Aspec
Primary Health Care

Aspects of Primary Health Care

2ND EDITION

KATHLEEN DENNILL • LAETITIA KING • TRINETTE SWANEPOEL

OXFORD
UNIVERSITY PRESS

OXFORD
UNIVERSITY PRESS

Great Clarendon Street, Oxford ox2 6DP

Oxford University Press is a department of the University of Oxford.
It further's the University's objective excellence in research, scholarship,
and education by publishing worldwide in

Oxford New York

Auckland Bangkok Buenos Aires Cape Town Chennai
Dar es Salaam Delhi Hong Kong Istanbul Karachi Kolkata
Kuala Lumpur Madrid Melbourne Mexico City Mumbai
Nairobi São Pualo Taipei Tokyo Toronto

Oxford is a registered trade mark of Oxford University Press
in the UK and certain other countries

Published in South Africa
by Oxford University Press Southern Africa, Cape Town

Aspects of Primary Health Care
Second edition
ISBN 0 19 571871 2

Previously published by Southern Book Publishers)Pty) Ltd
and by International Thomson Publishing Southern Africa (Pty) Ltd (1 86864 011 6)
First edition published 1995
Second edition published 1998
Tenth impression 2005

Cover design by Collage Graphics

Published by Oxford University Press Southern Africa
PO Box 12119, N1 City, 7463, Cape Town, South Africa

Set in 10 on 12.5 pt Palatino
Typesetting and reproduction by PG&A, Plumstead, Western Cape
Printed and bound by Paarl Print, Oosterland Street, Paarl, South Africa

Abridged Table of Contents

Contents

1

International views on primary health care

KATHLEEN DENNILL

"Health designates a process of adaption. It is not the result of instinct, but of an autonomous yet culturally shaped reaction to socially created reality." (Illich 1976 as quoted in Pritchard 1978:7)

CHAPTER OBJECTIVES

After reading this chapter, the student should be able to:

- explain what is understood by the concept of primary health care
- discuss the international development of primary health care as a means to obtain health for all by the year 2000 and beyond
- discuss different approaches to primary health care
- identify and use indicators to assess and plan for primary health care
- develop a successful strategy for the implementation of primary health care
- discuss trends in the global strategy of "health for all".

1.1 INTRODUCTION

The concept of primary health care developed in the 1940s and 1950s, when the governments of several countries were urged to rationalise their highly technical approach to health care and to broaden their coverage by providing better basic services that impact positively on health. In South Africa, two physicians, Drs Sidney and Emily Kark, started a health centre at Pholela in Zululand and developed a community-orientated primary care programme. This model proved so successful that by the end of the decade there were about 40 similar health centres in other rural areas. Despite publication about these and other successful programmes in international journals, these initiatives appear to have been regarded as irrelevant by other countries and by the newly constituted World Health Organisation (WHO).

1.2 ALMA-ATA

By the 1970s health care throughout the world was in turmoil, with fragmented health systems. The trend was towards expensive treatment for a few ill people rather than promotive and basic health care for many. These inequalities were found in both developed and developing countries world-wide.

In response to the international sense of despair at inadequate health care, an International Conference on Primary Health Care was jointly sponsored by the WHO and the United Nations Children's Fund (UNICEF). It was hosted by the government of the USSR at Alma-Ata from 6 to 12 September 1978. The conference was attended by 134 nations as well as many governmental and non-governmental organisations.

The primary health care philosophy introduced at this conference was endorsed with enthusiasm by the participating nations. It was seen as a means of achieving universally available health care and of attaining "health for all by the year 2000".

It had an immediate effect on the global strategies of the WHO and has dominated both its policies and programmes ever since. This conference has also had a substantial impact on the health policies of many nations, some with more success than others.

1.2.1 The concept of primary health care

The concept of primary health care encompasses a political philosophy that calls for radical changes in both the design and content of traditional health care services. It advocates an approach to health care based on principles that allow people to receive the care that enables them to lead socially and economically productive lives.

The definition of the concept as determined at Alma-Ata is:

> "Primary health care is essential care based on practical, scientifically sound and socially acceptable methods and technology, made universally accessible to individuals and families in the community through their full participation and at a cost that the community and country can afford to maintain at every stage of their development in the spirit of self-reliance and self-determination. It forms an integral part both of the country's health system, of which it is the central function and main focus, and of the overall social and economic development of the community. It is the first level of contact of individuals, the family and the community with the national health system, bringing health care as close as possible to where people live and work, and constitutes the first element of a continuing health care service." (WHO 1988:15)

The essential care aspect of primary health care consists of eight basic components (sometimes referred to as elements). These are listed under Section VII of the Declaration of Alma-Ata, which states that any primary health care programme should include at least these components.

The eight basic elements or components of primary health care are:

- education about prevailing health problems and methods of preventing and controlling them
- the promotion of food supply and proper nutrition
- an adequate supply of safe water and basic sanitation
- maternal and child health care, including family planning and care of high-risk groups
- immunisation against the major infectious diseases
- prevention and control of locally endemic diseases
- appropriate treatment of common diseases and injuries
- the provision of essential drugs.

Other components may and have been added to meet the specific needs identified by a community or country.

There is often confusion about what is understood by the concept of primary health care, as determined at Alma-Ata. The term is often used in texts and in practice to denote other meanings, therefore clarification is necessary:

- It is not primary care, primary medical care or primary curative care. Primary medical or curative care is the assessment (history-taking and physical examination) as well as specific care or treatment, of a client. Primary medical care is only one aspect of primary health care.
- It is not only first contact care. Primary health care services are the point of entry into the health system, but care can be ongoing until the problem is eradicated or the client is referred to a secondary service.
- It is not health services for all. Primary health care is more than health facilities and health personnel. It can only be successful if it is a part of community development. This requires a multidisciplinary team approach which co-ordinates all sectors involved in health and community development.
- It is not cheap, simple or second-class care. There is the misconception that hospital or high technology care is first-class medicine and that any other form of health care is second class. The success of primary health care lies in a comprehensive approach based on meeting the basic needs of the people which will enable them to live healthy lifestyles. The co-ordination and planning for this broad approach are complex, definitely not cheap and are based on the findings of scientific research which involves many disciplines, e.g. engineering, ecology and epidemiology.

Primary health care is the dynamic product of the community it serves, since it evolves from the economic, sociocultural and political characteristics of that community and is based on the needs identified by that community. The development of the health sector alone will not have a significant effect on the health of the people because many needs will not have been met.

A comprehensive approach to primary health care is therefore necessary to improve the health status of the community. This requires that health care be part of national political and economic strategies, and through this process the population should find access to employment opportunities and education, as well as better living and environmental conditions. This is an intersectoral and multidisciplinary approach to health care (see chapter 3).

Primary health care is therefore a broad concept, which is a combination of task-orientated basic health services and the process of community development.

1.2.2 The Declaration of Alma-Ata

At the conclusion of the conference a declaration of intent was drawn up. It sets out the principles and components in terms of which any primary health care service can be universally established.

DECLARATION OF ALMA-ATA

The International Conference on Primary Health Care, meeting in Alma-Ata this twelfth day of September in the year Nineteen hundred and seventy-eight, expressing the need for urgent action by all governments, all health and development workers, and the world community to protect and promote the health of all the people of the world, hereby makes the following Declaration:

I.
The Conference strongly reaffirms that health, which is a state of complete physical, mental and social wellbeing, and not merely the absence of disease or infirmity, is a fundamental human right and that the attainment of the highest possible level of health is a most important world-wide social goal whose realization requires the action of many other social and economic sectors in addition to the health sector.

II.
The existing gross inequality in the health status of the people, particularly between developed and developing countries as well as within countries, is politically, socially and economically unacceptable and is, therefore, of common concern to all countries.

III.
Economic and social development, based on a New International Economic Order, is of basic importance to the fullest attainment of health for all and to the reduction of the gap between the health status of the developing and developed countries. The promotion and protection of the health of the people is essential to sustained economic and social development and contributes to a better quality of life and to world peace.

IV.
The people have the right and duty to participate individually and collectively in the planning and implementation of their health care.

V.
Governments have a responsibility for the health of their people which can be fulfilled only by the provision of adequate health and social measures. A main social target of governments, international organizations and the whole world community in the coming decades should be

the attainment by all peoples of the world by the year 2000 of a level of health that will permit them to lead a socially and economically productive life. Primary health care is the key to attaining this target as part of development in the spirit of social justice.

VI.

Primary health care is essential health care based on practical, scientifically sound and socially acceptable methods and technology made universally accessible to individuals and families in the community through their full participation and at a cost that the community and country can afford to maintain at every stage of their development in the spirit of self-reliance and self-determination. It forms an integral part both of the country's health system, of which it is the central function and main focus, and of the overall social and economic development of the community. It is the first level of contact of individuals, the family and community with the national health system, bringing health care as close as possible to where people live and work, and constitutes the first element of a continuing health care process.

VII.

Primary health care:

1. reflects and evolves from the economic conditions and sociocultural and political characteristics of the country and its communities and is based on the application of the relevant results of social, biomedical and health services research and public health experience;
2. addresses the main health problems in the community, providing promotive, preventive, curative and rehabilitative services accordingly;
3. includes at least: education concerning prevailing health problems and the methods of preventing and controlling them; promotion of food supply and proper nutrition; an adequate supply of safe water and basic sanitation; maternal and child health care, including family planning; immunization against the major infectious diseases; prevention and control of locally endemic diseases; appropriate treatment of common diseases and injuries; and provision of essential drugs;
4. involves, in addition to the health sector, all related sectors and aspects of national and community development, in particular agriculture, animal husbandry, food, industry, education, housing, public works, communications and other sectors; and demands the coordinated efforts of all those sectors;
5. requires and promotes maximum community and individual self-reliance and participation in the planning, organization, operation and control of primary health care, making fullest use of local, national and other available resources; and to this end develops through appropriate education the ability of communities to participate;
6. should be sustained by integrated, functional and mutually-supportive referral systems, leading to the progressive improvement of comprehensive health care for all, and giving priority to those most in need;
7. relies, at local and referral levels, on health workers, including physicians, nurses, midwives, auxiliaries and community workers as applicable, as well as traditional practitioners as needed, suitably trained socially and technically to work as a health team and to respond to the expressed health needs of the community.

VIII.

All governments should formulate national policies, strategies and plans of action to launch and sustain primary health care as part of a comprehensive national health system and in coordination with other sectors. To this end, it will be necessary to exercise political will, to mobilize the country's resources and to use available external resources rationally.

IX.

All countries should cooperate in a spirit of partnership and service to ensure primary health care for all people, since the attainment of health by people in any one country directly concerns and benefits every other country. In this context the joint WHO/UNICEF report on primary health care constitutes a solid basis for the further development and operation of primary health care throughout the world.

X.

An acceptable level of health for all the people of the world by the year 2000 can be attained through a fuller and better use of the world's resources, a considerable part of which is now spent on armaments and military conflicts. A genuine policy of independence, peace, détente and disarmament could and should release additional resources that could well be devoted to peaceful aims and in particular to the acceleration of social and economic development of which primary health care, as an essential part, should be allotted its proper share.

Source: WHO (1978:428–30)

1.2.3 Strategy for the implementation of primary health care

For a strategy to be determined, first and foremost there must be political commitment to primary health care by the government in power. Priorities must be identified and then detailed plans of action must be set out. This will vary from country to country, depending on its level of development, health needs and available resources. Most health systems need to be adapted to a more community-based or decentralised system, so that services become available to all.

(a) Principles on which a successful strategy should be based

A successful strategy for implementing primary health care chould be based on the following:

- *Equity.* All people should have equal access to basic health care and social services. There should be an absence of any subgroup variability and discrepancy in care.
- *Accessibility.* Services must be extended to be within the reach of all people in the country. Special attention must be given to disadvantaged regions of the country, especially small isolated rural areas. Services must be:
  - geographically accessible, meaning that health services should be within a reasonable distance (the WHO suggests 5-10 km) and that transport should be available
  - financially accessible to the individual and the community
  - functionally accessible, in that the appropriate type of care be available to meet the needs of the specific community.
- *Affordability.* The level of health care offered should be aligned to what the community and the country can afford. No person should be denied health care because of an inability to pay.
- *Availability.* There should be sufficient and appropriate services to meet the particular health needs of each community.

- *Effectiveness.* The services provided must do what they were intended to do for the specific community. The effectiveness of the service must also be justifiable in terms of total cost.
- *Efficiency.* The results attained should be proportionate to the input, in terms of effort expended, money spent, resources used and time utilised.

(b) Reorganisation of health services

A shift in the emphasis of health care is necessary, from curative hospital-based care to community-based primary health care. The overall objective is to deliver health services efficiently and effectively through an infrastructure that covers the needs of communities at ground or district levels, with the necessary support and referral services at intermediate or provincial level and at central or national level. This process of change needs to be dynamic, as it will be influenced by the political, cultural, technical and financial factors of the country. It will also require the realignment of available resources to meet this new structure, with a shift of resources going to the community for community-based health care and basic health services. Problems arise when government bureaucracies look for easily manageable and replicable interventions to introduce across the whole country or province at community level.

This does not allow for the flexible and adaptive approach necessary for the implementation of appropriate primary health care services to meet the needs of each community. To counteract this problem, much more autonomy should be given to the people of each community to assess their own health needs and determine how to plan their own primary health care services to meet these needs. The success of primary health care depends to a large degree on the community "ownership" of its health services.

(c) Multidisciplinary approach

The definition of health contained in the constitution of the WHO acknowledges the broader dimensions of health. It states that health is the ... "physical, mental and social well-being, and not merely the absence of disease and infirmity". It can therefore be said that health is the product of a person's positive interaction with his or her total environment. The aspects of this holistic approach towards attaining what people refer to as health, are well illustrated in the mandala of health (Figure 1.2.) The traditional health team who are involved in health care delivery cannot attain this goal on their own. According to King (1996:23), the multidisciplinary team must include "the ordinary individual in the community, be it the patient and his family, or any other concerned individual or group that can assist the community in one way or another towards the improvement of their health status" (see chapter 3).

FIGURE 1.1: Health care hierarchy

The typical or traditional pyramid:

The doctor is at the top and health care is mostly institution-based

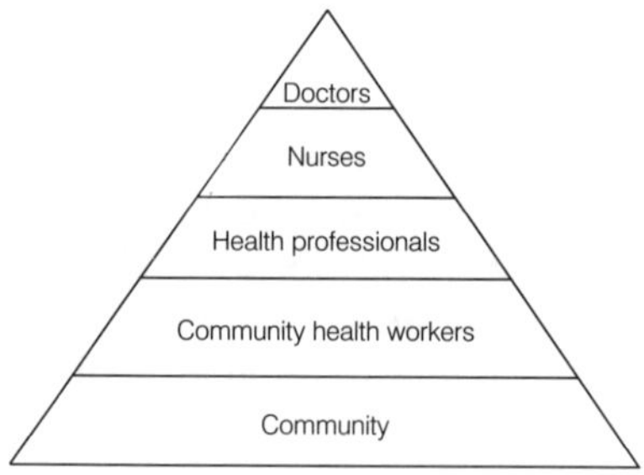

The community is at the bottom and has little input into the health care it receives

The pyramid as it should be:

Primary health care is community-based

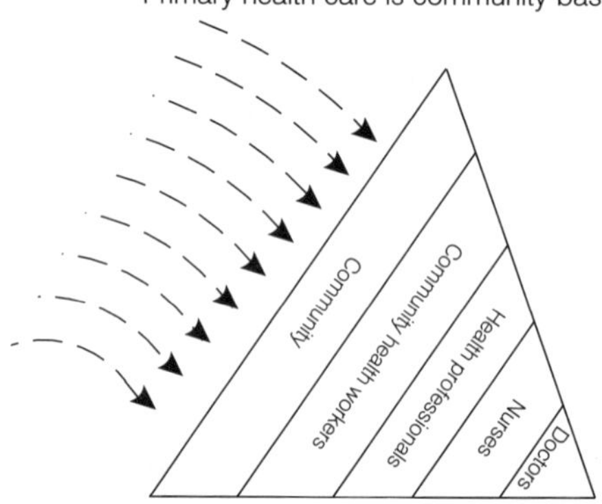

The community is an equal partner with all other participating health workers, including health professionals

(d) Intersectoral collaboration

Primary health care includes such diverse interventions that it cannot be implemented by health workers alone. Different sectors have the different resources, skills and technology necessary for the attainment of a healthy community. It is said that civil engineers have a greater effect on the health of people than health professionals, because of the part they play in supplying the community with safe water and sanitation.

FIGURE 1.2: The mandala of health – a model of the human ecosystem

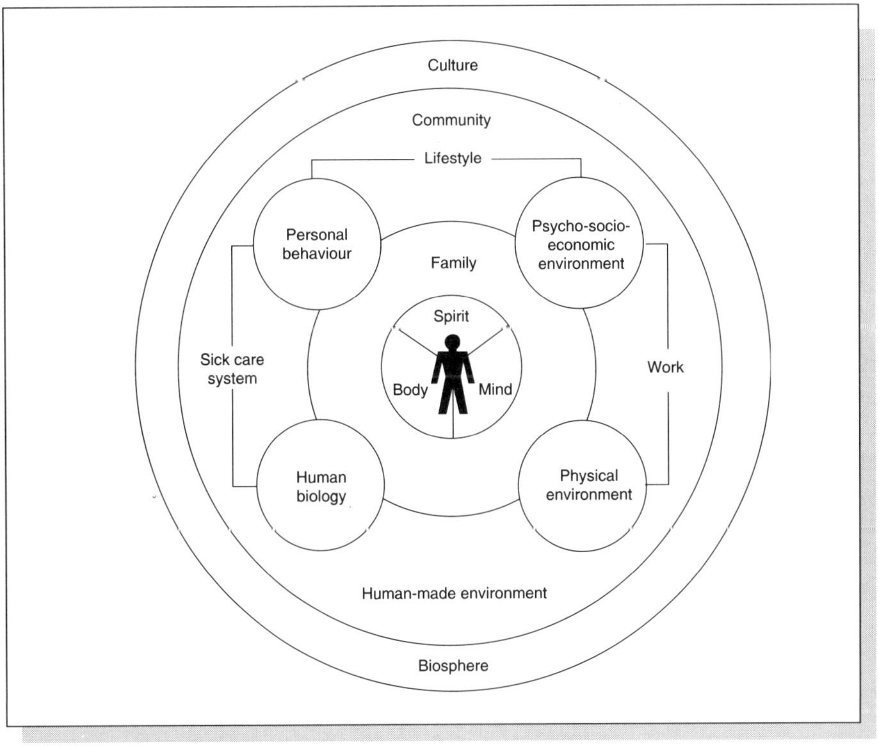

Source: Gilbert *et al.* (1996:8)

There should be multisectoral input in determining policy which impacts on health or the environment. For example, the health of a community can be affected both beneficially and adversely by the building of a large dam in their area. To enhance the benefit of such a project to the community, a team approach by the different sectors or role-players in the project (e.g. from health, engineering, ecology disciplines, etc.) is required (see chapter 3).

(e) Community participation and involvement

This is a shift of emphasis, from external agencies supplying the health services, to the people of the community becoming active participants in their own health care. They become partners in health care by generating their own ideas, assessing their needs, making decisions, planning, implementing and even evaluating the care they receive. This process encourages and allows the community to take responsibility for their own situation, thus empowering them. It encourages community development of self-reliance and self-determination (see chapter 3).

Since Alma-Ata, the concept of primary health care has evolved and changed. Three of the most important international events that have influenced and changed the development of primary health care programmes around the world will be discussed. They are GOBI-FFF, the Ottawa Charter and the Riga Conference.

1.3 GOBI-FFF

Three years after Alma-Ata the United Nations Children's Fund (UNICEF) announced the launch of the programme called the "Child survival development revolution". The objective of the programme was to counteract the high morbidity and mortality of infants and children in the developing world. UNICEF published a report of findings which demonstrated that the improvement in the welfare of children was very limited despite the introduction of primary health care. Infant mortality rates had fallen steadily in the 1960s and early 1970s, but in the later 1970s, around the time of Alma-Ata, the rates hardly changed. The report further claimed that primary health care as envisaged at Alma-Ata was too costly and would take too long to implement. The "revolution" that was suggested to hasten the process was based on a widespread adoption of cheap, easy, accessible and simple technologies. These were directed at those conditions responsible for a large proportion of infant and child morbidity and mortality. The four activities that were recommended to accomplish this were:

- G–growth monitoring using child growth charts
- O–oral rehydration
- B–promotion of breast-feeding
- I–expanded immunisation.

In 1984 UNICEF, WHO and other interested parties met at Bellagio to promote these activities. It was recommended that the emphasis first be placed on the immunisation phase of the programme. This would be followed by oral rehydration and the other phases as soon as possible.

At this meeting three more activities were added to the other recommendations:

- F–food supplementation
- F–female literacy
- F–family planning.

This programme was widely criticised, since it selected certain groups within the community for specific interventions and was a move away from the original broad comprehensive approach to primary health care. Despite this controversy GOBI-FFF has been almost universally accepted as a part of primary health care. Each intervention will be discussed briefly.

1.3.1 Growth monitoring

Regular monitoring of the growth of a child during the first five years of its life allows the nutritional status to be assessed. Height and mass are recorded on the individual's growth chart against his or her age, which is then compared to the standard curves printed on the card representing international norms. A steady increase in the height and mass of the child will usually indicate good health, while an abnormal or insufficient mass gain will indicate a level of malnutrition and can be associated with increased risks to other conditions and infections.

1.3.2 Oral rehydration therapy

An estimated four to five million children die each year from dehydration, usually as a result of diarrhoea. Teaching mothers how to make and administer a simple fluid replacement solution of boiled water, salt and sugar, can save many lives. Replacement fluid is made from one litre of boiled water, to which one teaspoon of salt and eight teaspoons of sugar are added.

1.3.3 Breast-feeding

Breast-feeding must be promoted as "breast is best" for infant health. Besides the cost benefits, mother's milk is more nutritious and imparts immunity to the infant against infection. An additional benefit is that it does offer some protection to mothers against falling pregnant, because lactation suppresses ovulation. This is of paramount importance in reducing infant and maternal mortality rates in developing countries.

1.3.4 Immunisation

Immunisation is a low-cost way of reducing mortality rates in children under five. In developing countries approximately five million children die per annum from conditions against which they can be immunised. The WHO has introduced a successful programme called the Expanded Programme on Immunisation (EPI), to protect children against the major infectious diseases – measles, polio, diphtheria, pertussis, neonatal tetanus, tuberculosis and yellow fever. This programme has proved very successful in participating countries.

1.3.5 Food supplementation

This refers to feeding schemes used to supplement the deficient diets of people due to the effects of famine or poverty. It also refers to weaning foods which are introduced to the infant's diet when it requires more than just mother's milk. The teaching of food gardening, or subsistence farming, diet planning and healthy methods of cooking are also part of this intervention.

1.3.6 Female literacy

There is a correlation in developing countries between low female literacy rates and high infant and maternal mortality rates. Studies have shown that literacy can empower a mother by enabling her to make informed choices that enhance both her own and her child's health.

1.3.7 Family planning

Women should be taught that they have a choice as to how many children they have and when they have them. Since mothers are usually the care-givers, this knowledge empowers them to make decisions that will affect both their own health and that of their children.

1.3.8 Conclusion

An additional F has been added by some countries for first-aid.

At the conclusion of the Bellagio meeting a consensus report was prepared, which concluded: "primary health care should respond to all of the health needs of the community, but priority should be given to those interventions that will rapidly reduce mortality and morbidity at the least possible cost." (Walsh and Warren 1986:ix)

1.4 OTTAWA CHARTER

A conference on health promotion was held in Ottawa on 21 November 1986 to focus on the goal to achieve "health for all" by the year 2000. The objective was to look at the health promotion aspect of primary health care and through this determine means which would enable people to increase control over, and to improve, their health. To a large extent the Declaration of Alma-Ata had failed to address this aspect of health care, but the WHO had established a programme in Europe on health promotion in 1984.

FIGURE 1.3: The effect of the environment on health

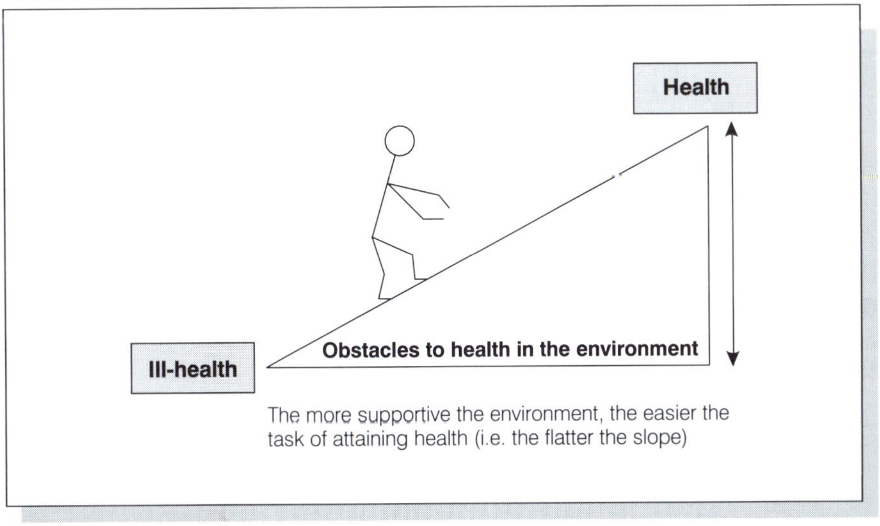

Health is defined by the WHO as "a state of complete physical, mental and social well-being". To reach this state, people must be enabled to realise aspirations, satisfy basic needs and change or cope with the environment. The charter gives the following key points as a means to attain this state:

- *Build public policies that support health.* Health promotion must go beyond health care by making health care an agenda item for all policy-makers. It requires that obstacles to health-promoting policies be identified in non-medical sectors and that ways be found to remove them. The aim is to ensure safer and health-orientated public services.
- *Create supportive environments.* At both a global and local level, health is influenced by the way in which we treat our environment. Communities which exploit the environment without attention to the ecology will reap the effects of ill health as well as social problems, because that environment will not be able to support them. Through health promotion, living and working conditions can be created that are safe and pleasant.
- *Strengthen community action.* For health promotion to be successful, communities must be empowered and have control over their own initiatives and activities. They must draw on their own human and material resources in the community to enhance self-help and social support. Health professionals must learn to work with communities.
- *Develop personal skills.* Personal and social development must be enhanced by providing health information and health education to help people develop the skills they need to make healthy choices. This should enable people to prepare themselves for the different stages of life as well

as for chronic illness or injuries, should they occur. This preparation should take place in schools, at home, at work and in community settings.

- *Reorientate health services.* The responsibility for health promotion must be shared by individuals, health professionals, community groups, health service institutions and government departments. This requires that the health sector move beyond the provision of clinical and curative services, to a health promotion approach sensitive to cultural differences.

Health promotion is therefore a multifaceted approach for the prevention of ill health. This approach includes strategies such as education, community development, mass communication, self-help, public policy development and even organisational change (Wardrop 1993:34). Health promotion therefore advocates social as well as individual responsibility for health and is a vital part of primary health care.

1.5 RIGA

A meeting was held at Riga, USSR, from 22 to 25 March 1988, to renew and strengthen commitments to "health for all by the year 2000, a midpoint perspective". It brought together experts from all regions of the WHO, UNICEF, United Nations Development Programme (UNDP) and non-governmental organisations.

Progress was evident in that many national health systems had been restructured to provide comprehensive primary health care. There was an increase in the equality and effectiveness of health services but the gains were not uniform between countries or even within a country.

In many developing countries immunisation rates had risen and there was a decrease in infant, under-five and maternal mortality rates. Unfortunately many of the least developed areas lacked the political commitment and other resources necessary and as a result had made little progress.

Other problems, such as massive urbanisation and population growth, had occurred in many of these countries. This resulted in widespread poverty and the overloading of available resources, which had a detrimental effect on the health of people.

To address the persisting and emerging problems which were evident in many participating countries, delegates determined to renew and adapt commitments made at Alma-Ata.

Resolutions were adopted to assist and motivate them, including the following:

- *Maintaining health for all as a permanent goal of all nations up to and beyond the year 2000.* The goal of health for all would stay the same but problems would develop and change over time, from country to country and also from community to community within a country. The principles underlying primary health care would remain - equality, effectiveness, affordability, community participation and intersectoral collaboration. Problems would change so the methods of dealing with them would also have to change.

- *Renewing and strengthening strategies for health for all.* Each country should continue to monitor its own health problems, identify its most seriously underserved and vulnerable populations and develop its own strategies to deal with them. Development and implementation of these strategies would invite active participation from the people affected.
- *Intensifying social and political action for health.* Political and social commitment are prerequisites for the success of primary health care programmes. The value of political commitment is limited if it is not supported by the necessary finances and structural rearrangements, the appropriate policies and adequate leadership. Social action needs support from individual citizens, groups of people in the community and national and international organisations. The WHO committed itself to both a leadership and supporting role in this endeavour.
- *Developing and mobilising leadership for health for all.* The quality of leadership and the availability of sufficient leaders is vital to the success of primary health care programmes. Leaders must be trained and developed at community, district and national levels to meet this challenge.
- *Empowering people.* Improvement in the health status of people at community level depends to a large extent on their decisions. Empower people to make the correct decisions, by providing them with the necessary information and the technical support which will enable them to share in opportunities and take responsibility regarding their own health.
- *Making intersectoral collaboration a force for health for all.* Health is not the responsibility of the health sector alone. It is dependent on the social and financial involvement of both government and non-government institutions. Adequate clean water and sanitation, improved housing, education, agriculture and a sustainable ecology, are all factors which impact on health. Intersectoral collaboration is therefore a must, if health for all is to be attained.
- *Strengthening district health services based on primary health care.* District or decentralised health services are necessary to achieve coverage at community level. This allows adaptation to local needs and the targeting of specific problems, while maintaining an effective infrastructure. The success of such a service is, however, dependent on an adequate and suitable referral system to higher, more complex levels of care.
- *Planning, preparing and supporting health personnel for health for all.* The education and training of health personnel at all levels need reorientation

to address community-based health problems. Better management practices, personnel support systems and incentives to encourage and maintain motivated health workers, must be developed for those working in difficult and often remote locations.

- *Ensuring the development and rational use of science and appropriate technology.* Research must be encouraged to supply the necessary information and develop the appropriate technology to improve the health of the most deprived people. As areas develop, so will their demand for more advanced technology increase.
- *Overcoming problems that continue to resist solution.* In many of the least developed countries of the world, the people are the victims of their lack of development. The situation is one that is almost impossible for the country itself to address. Population growth continues at abnormally high levels, infant and maternal mortality rates are unacceptable and the environmental resources are overtaxed, with the resulting negative effect on the health of the people. In order to confront this situation the WHO, with its member countries, will have to commit themselves to help these countries develop. The help required will include both technical and physical resources.

At the conclusion of the conference the following statement summed up the situation (WHO 1988:62):

> "As WHO turns the corner of the first decade after Alma-Ata, it needs to ready itself to face a new set of problems. In particular, it must appreciate that tomorrow will not be yesterday, and that yesterday's answers, though they brought glory, will not serve tomorrow."

1.6 APPROACHES TO PRIMARY HEALTH CARE

1.6.1 Comprehensive versus selective primary health care

One year after Alma-Ata and the launch of primary health care as a comprehensive approach to attain "health for all" by the year 2000, Walsh and Warren (1979) threw the cat among the pigeons by presenting a paper under the title of "Selective primary health care: an interim strategy for disease control in developing countries". It advocated an approach that was problem-orientated and cost-effective.

The implementation of selective primary health care programmes is relatively easy and inexpensive. These programmes are attractive to funders, since results can usually be statistically or quantifiably measured in a relatively short period of time. These selective primary health care programmes have a "success" factor which has made them popular with international health organisations, despite their commitment to comprehensive health care.

UNICEF's GOBI-FFF campaign, the WHO's Expanded Programme on Immunisation (EPI) and the Control of Diarrhoeal Diseases (CDD), which emphasises oral rehydration, are all examples of selective primary health care.

Selective primary health care is concerned with medical interventions or effective technologies which can be implemented anywhere and are aimed at improving the health status of many individuals at the lowest cost.

Comprehensive primary health care, on the other hand, is not an alternative to health care delivery, it is a strategy for the health development of a community. The emphasis of these comprehensive programmes is on change in the community rather than on a programme which can be replicated and instituted in any community.

Banerji (in Rifkin and Walt 1986:560) questioned the selective approach for the following reasons:

- It gives a large proportion of resource allocations to people with priority diseases or conditions only.
- It reinforces authoritarian attitudes rather than community participation.
- It has a questionable moral and ethical value, since some designated interest groups overrule the majority of the people.
- It has a fragile scientific basis.

This selective approach is palliative in nature, dealing in the management of identified health problems. McDonald (1993:11) says that "... selective primary health care can be seen as a refusal of the medical world to accept the challenge of comprehensive primary health care and to incorporate it into existing ways of thinking and doing". Health care should deal with "the physical, mental and social well-being of the individual" (WHO 1978:2). The selective approach opposes the principle of equitability in primary health care and also excludes the effect of environmental and economic factors on health. It does, however, save lives and is community-based rather than institution-based.

Mosley (1988:907–8) felt there was a middle way in primary health care, one that emphasised the problem-orientated approach in preference to the technology-orientated or disease-orientated approach. He introduced a new concept to primary health care, that of "categorical programmes" This problem-orientated approach defines a series of tasks or strategies that are focused and manageable. Primary health care can be directed towards a disease such as malaria as well as to more general health problems such as a poor environment or a high infant mortality rate. This would require both an intersectoral approach and community involvement - a comprehensive approach.

In some literature the term "selective" is sometimes interchanged with "vertical" and the term "comprehensive" with "horizontal" when referring to primary health care programmes.

1.6.2 Microscopic versus macroscopic or medical versus health model

The microscopic approach is where the focus of both efforts and resources is on the curative side of health care and the patient is a passive recipient. McKeown likened the Western medical model to an engineering model, where the body is a machine and the medical professional the scientist who intervenes to find and treat a disorder. The person's problem was treated with no reference to the community or to the environment in which the person lives. In his book McKeown (1976:65) showed that diseases such as tuberculosis and measles (see Figure 1.4) were controlled through improving the environment rather than through medical treatment such as chemotherapy and vaccination.

People are part of a wider system such as the family or community. This interaction with other people and with the environment in which people find themselves will affect their health. This is a holistic approach that is sometimes referred to as an outward or macroscopic approach. The emphasis here is to create an environment and promote lifestyles which prevent the body from breaking down. This is known as the health model.

An analogy of a river has been used into which the medical practitioner has to constantly dive to rescue people as they are carried in the river of ill health. He or she is so busy doing this that there is no time to determine how all these persons landed in the river, or to go upstream to stop the person who is pushing them in! We need to move to a health model that emphasises prevention rather than cure.

In comprehensive primary health care there is room for both approaches but the macroscopic approach or health model must be emphasised (MacDonald 1993:41–4).

1.7 INDICATORS

Indicators are methods used at regional, national and international levels to plan and evaluate health care programmes. As the name suggests, they are an indication or reflection of a given situation. They can be defined as variables which help to measure change (WHO 1981:12).

Information is required in order to determine these indicators and for this purpose data need to be collected and analysed. They are important to primary health care because they will indicate the success or failure of programmes, as well as give direction to planners to develop the necessary services required to meet the needs of individuals and community.

To be valid, the indicator must measure what it is supposed to measure, while to be reliable, the results should be the same if measured by different people, at different times and under different circumstances.

FIGURE 1.4: McKeown graph: death rate from measles of children under 15 in England and Wales

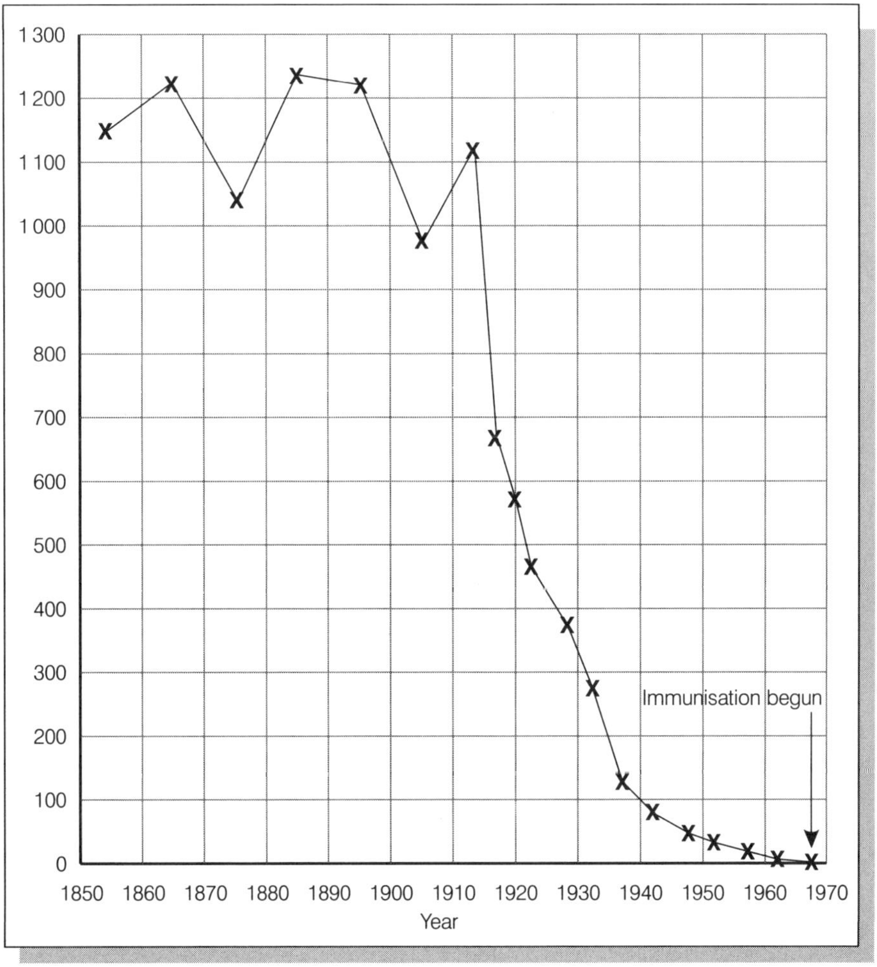

Source: McKeown (1976)

1.7.1 Sources of data

For the successful use of indicators, a reliable and accessible information system is required, since the indicator is only as useful as the accuracy of the information on which it is based. Sources of data commonly used include:

- vital events registers, such as birth and death registers
- population and housing censuses
- routine health service records

- disease registers
- epidemiological surveillance data
- surveys.

Data from the non-health sector can also be included.

1.7.2 Global indicators

The WHO has identified global indicators against which countries can assess their progress in attaining "health for all". By determining the number of countries that have attained these goals, the success of primary health care as a global strategy, can be evaluated. The following are some of the more common global indicators used:

- At least 5% of the Gross National Product of a country is to be spent on health.
- Resources must be equitably distributed.
- Safe water is to be available in the home or within 15 minutes' walking distance.
- Local health care services should be within one hour's walking distance and have at least 20 essential drugs available.
- The nutritional status of children should be adequate, with
  - 90% of newborn infants attaining a birth weight of at least 2 500 g
  - 90% of children registering a weight for age that corresponds to the reference values.
- The infant mortality rate to be below 50 per 1 000 live births.
- Life expectancy at birth to be over 60 years.
- The adult literacy rate is to exceed 70%.
- The Gross National Product per capita is to exceed US$ 500 per annum.

1.7.3 Categories of indicators

The WHO has provided a list from which countries can choose the indicators which are most relevant to their health needs and socio-economic situations. There are four categories of indicators:

- health policy indicators
- social and economic indicators
- indicators of the provision of health care
- indicators of health status.

(a) Health policy indicators

- *Political commitment.* This is difficult to measure but usually takes the form of a policy statement in favour of health for all or a health charter which is issued by the highest level of political authority in the country.

- *Resource allocation.* The government transfers its declaration of intent into a budget as it allocates resources to health. The proportion of the Gross National Product (GNP) spent on health and that spent on related activities such as education, housing, water supply and nutrition, are good indicators. The amount of the health budget spent on primary health care is also of importance.
- *The degree of equality of distribution of health resources.* The indicators of importance here are the distribution of per capita expenditure from area to area; the proportion of total expenditure going to primary health care per region and the ratios of hospital beds and health workers to populations in different areas.
- *Community involvement.* This is difficult to measure, but can to a limited degree be assessed by the degree of decentralisation in decision-making that occurs. Another indicator is the number of ways that people have to express their demands and needs through political means or groups like trade unions and women's organisations.
- *Organisational framework and managerial process.* Is there interdepartmental, interorganisational and intersectoral communication as well as collaboration in management to ensure an adequate and integrated primary health care service?

(b) Social and economic indicators

- *Rate of population growth.* Demographic factors such as the size and the rate of natural increase of the population, as well as the age and sex distribution, are important for health planning. Birth, mortality and fertility rates are also important indicators, especially in assessing the success of programmes.
- *Gross national product or gross domestic product per capita.* To determine this, the total gross national or domestic product is divided by the total population of the country to give an average income level. This will give an indication of the general welfare of the people in a country. This is usually an indicator which applies to the whole country and is rarely calculable for districts or communities. The annual World Bank Atlas has this information available as a global indicator.
- *Income distribution.* This is a less reliable indicator because it is not usually determined annually and is often ambiguous or incorrect. Income information is usually collected during a national population census or by a household survey in a specific area.
- *Working conditions.* Indicators which are of value here include levels of

unemployment and the percentage of groups such as women or disabled people employed. The number of dependent persons, either under 15 or over 65, is also of importance because it indicates the number of people in a community who do not have an earning capacity.

- *Adult literacy rate.* This is assessed by identifying the number of people 15 years and over who are able to read and write. The actual rate is difficult to determine since it depends on self-reporting. However, it is of particular importance, especially when applied to women. The woman in the home provides basic health care and being literate allows her a wider understanding of health issues and empowers her to make better informed decisions. Also of importance here are statistics on education, such as the proportion of children at school, the amount per capita spent on education and the ratio of children per teacher.
- *Housing.* The adequacy of housing is usually determined by the national population census, and is based on the number of persons per room. The proportion of the population in informal housing is also an indicator.
- *Food availability.* This is based on the availability of food at national level as determined by local food production, exports and imports. This is a national indicator, while local conditions and seasonal variations must be taken into account.

(c) Indicators of the provision of health care

- *Coverage by primary health care.* The distance of people from the nearest health service is an indicator. The WHO suggests the distance should not be more than 10 km. The indicators here relate to the eight essential components or elements of primary health care:
  - People's understanding of common health problems and methods of preventing and controlling them are difficult to measure. This can be done by community surveys but these do not measure attitudinal or behavioural changes. Another indicator is the number of hours coverage given by the mass media to health information (i.e. radio, television and newspapers).
  - Food and nutrition indicators have already been discussed.
  - The percentage of the population of the country or a community who have access to safe water and adequate sanitation facilities is an important indicator.
  - The level of maternal and child care can be assessed by fertility and birth rates as well as by the intervals between births. Also of importance is the accessibility and use of available services such as antenatal care, baby clinics, family planning, etc.

- Immunisation is determined by assessing the percentage of children at risk who are fully immunised. The objective is to obtain an immunisation level of 80% or more.
- The control of endemic diseases is not easy to assess, except for those diseases which are notifiable. However, a study could be done in a certain area to determine a condition such as the incidence of diarrhoea and could also determine the use of oral rehydration.
- Essential drugs should be available at the primary health care service whenever required. Periodic surveys can be done to assess this.

- *Coverage by the referral system.* For primary health care to be successful, it is necessary to have adequate and appropriate referral facilities. The emergency referral facility should be no further than two hours away by road. The proportion of the population within this range can be determined. The ratios of various categories of health worker per the population is also a valuable indicator.

(d) Indicators of health status

The following statistics are of importance (WHO 1981(b):9–40 and El Bendari-Hammond and Smith 1992:46,148):

- infant mortality rate
- child mortality rate
- life expectancy
- maternal mortality rate
- morbidity (usually given as the incidence or prevalence rate).

When selecting indicators to monitor the progress of a health programme, select a few indicators rather than many and choose them so that they have social and political punch, in the sense that people and policy-makers will be motivated into action by them. The indicators selected must also be appropriate to the means available for data collection.

For the successful use of indicators in primary health care, an effective information system at every level of management must be established and maintained. The World Bank has supported over 260 projects in 63 countries with information technology components since Alma-Ata. This information technology can include a combination of computer technology, micro-electronic applications, information systems, communication techniques and methods. This type of system processes the data that have been collected into usable information in a relatively short period of time and has been successfully implemented in developing countries like India and Uganda. Having this data processed and fed back into the system quickly allows for informed decision-making based on constantly changing health conditions.

This, in turn, results in the available resources being optimally used for the benefit of the community served.

1.8 TRENDS IN THE GLOBAL STRATEGY OF PRIMARY HEALTH CARE

Through the process of implementing primary health care, trends have become evident in various spheres.

1.8.1 Developed countries

Many of these countries have made substantial progress in bringing health services to their people. An ageing population has emerged in these countries because of an increased life expectancy, resulting in a shift in health problems to more chronic conditions. Rapid urbanisation has also affected health needs, with problems related to new lifestyles, high-risk behaviour and deteriorating environments. The emphasis of the services in these countries is to meet these new needs and to reduce socio-economic disparities. The global economic downturn has meant there is less to spend on health.

1.8.2 Developing countries

Many of these countries have made significant progress in establishing a health infrastructure based on primary health care. As the programme evolves and needs are met, new health needs emerge, similar to those mentioned above, which need to be addressed, often with diminishing resources.

Some developing countries continue to struggle with very high infant and maternal mortality rates and alarming morbidity rates. Socio-economic conditions are poor, resources are scarce and to date there has been a lack of political backing for primary health care, or the philosophy is misunderstood. The situations are often compounded by natural and man-made disasters. These countries require both technical and financial support from the international community to aid them in their national development and health policies if optimal health is to be attained.

1.8.3 The multidisciplinary primary health care team

According to IJsselmuiden (1993:68) the current training of health workers is largely compartmentalised and therefore inappropriate for the multidisciplinary approach needed to implement primary health care successfully. Although there are successful initiatives in training health professionals at a post basic qualification level, such as the schools of public health, there is a need to place greater emphasis on the multidisciplinary team concept in the basic training of all the health team members.

Nurses are the most universal members of the multidisciplinary primary health care team. To function effectively in primary health care, nurses have identified the need for special preparation. Skills, including clinical skills, need to be adapted and added to existing training, to give a more dynamic shape to nursing practice in the community.

In-service and multidisciplinary training must be ongoing, to allow the team members to acquire the dynamic skills needed to meet the unique requirements of communities. Legal barriers and other constraints affecting the team member's contribution must be addressed, so that optimal use of each team member's skills can be made.

1.8.4 Cultural sensitivity

The cultural and ethnic diversity found both globally and within countries has been acknowledged. Appropriate primary health care interventions should be planned with sensitivity to the beliefs, values and social networks of each specific community. To accomplish this, members of the health team must become culturally aware and must encourage input from the community to identify their own felt needs. Programmes that have been found to be successful are those that are acceptable and appropriate to the community.

1.9 SUMMARY

The substantial gains in health and in the pursuit of health care for all over the last 22 years have reaffirmed the validity of the declaration of Alma-Ata for all countries, at all stages of development. In the implementation of primary health care, conflicts of interest have occurred between the new strategies and the existing organisational structures and management. Since the primary health care strategy is not negotiable, ways to facilitate structural changes in health systems and develop suitable management need to be identified and implemented. Some of the less developed countries are finding it difficult to sustain and evaluate their programmes; help must be given by those countries with the necessary expertise. The struggling global economy and the emergence of the AIDS pandemic are also factors that have slowed the progress and changed the path of primary health care. The goal of health care available to all remains the objective. However, the time frame will need to extend beyond the year 2000.

Bibliography

Bergerhoff, P., Lehmann, D. and Novak, P. (Eds) 1990. *Primary health care: public involvement, family medicine and health economics.* Berlin: Springer-Verlag.

Coreil, J. and Mull, J.D. 1990. *Anthropology and primary health care.* Boulder: Westview Press.

Cork, M. 1990. Approaches to health promotion. *Midwife, health visitor and community nurse.* Vol. 26, No. 5.

El Bindari-Hammond, A. and Smith, D.L. 1992. *Primary health care reviews: guidelines and methods.* Geneva: WHO.

Gilbert, L., Selikow, T. and Walker, L. 1996. *Society, health and disease: An introductory reader for health professionals.* Randburg: Ravan.

IJsselmuiden, C. 1993. The Transvaal School of Public Health: towards education for health.*CHASA journal of comprehensive health.* Vol. 4, No. 3:57–61.

King, L.J. 1996. Community participation in health care delivery: a nursing perspective. DLitt et Phil. Pretoria: University of South Africa.

MacDonald, J.J. 1993. *Primary health care: medicine in its place.* London: Earthscan.

McCloskey, J.C. and Grace, H.K. 1990. *Current issues in nursing.* St Louis: Mosby.

McMurray, A. 1990. *Community health nursing: primary health care in practice.* Melbourne: Churchill Livingstone.

McKeown, T. 1976. *The role of medicine: dream, mirage or nemesis?* London: Nuffield Provincial Hospitals' Trust.

Morgan, R.E. and Rau, B. 1993. *Global learning for health.* Washington DC: National Council for International Health.

Mosley, W.H. 1988. Is there a middle way? Categorical programmes for primary health care. *Social science medicine.* Vol. 9, No. 9:907–8.

Phillips, D.R. 1990. *Health and health care in the Third World.* New York: Longman.

Pritchard, P. 1978. *Manual of primary health care: its nature and organisation.* Oxford: Oxford University Press.

Rifkin, S.B. and Walt, G. 1986. Why health improves: defining the issues concerning "Comprehensive primary health care" and "Selective primary health care". *Social science medicine.* Vol. 23, No. 6:559–66.

Streefland, P. and Charbot, J. (Eds) 1990. *Implementing primary health care.* Amsterdam: Royal Tropical Institute.

Walsh, J.A. and Warren, K.S. 1979. Selective primary health care: an interim strategy for disease control in developing countries. *New England journal of medicine.* Vol. 301:967–74.

Walsh, J.A. and Warren, K.S. (Eds) 1986. *Strategies for primary health care –*

technologies appropriate for the control of disease in the developing world. Chicago: University of Chicago Press.

Wardrop, K. 1993. A framework for health promotion. *Canadian journal of public health.* Vol. 84, Supplement 1.

Wilson, R.G., Bryant, J.H., Echols, B.E. and Abrantes, A. (Eds) 1988. *Management information systems and microcomputers in primary health care.* Geneva: Aga Khan Foundation.

Wisner, B. 1987. GOBI versus PHC? Some dangers of selective primary health care. *Social science medicine.* Vol. 24, No. 1:1–7.

World Health Organisation. 1978. The Alma-Ata conference on primary health care. *WHO chronicle,* Vol. 32:409–30.

World Health Organisation. 1981(a). *Global strategy for health for all by the year 2000.* Geneva: WHO.

World Health Organisation. 1981(b). *Development of indicators for monitoring progress towards health for all by the year 2000.* Geneva: WHO.

World Health Organisation. 1986. *Regulatory mechanisms for nursing training and practice: meeting primary health care needs.* Geneva: WHO.

World Health Organisation. 1987. *Eighth general programme of work – covering the period 1990–1995.* Geneva: WHO.

World Health Organisation. 1988. *From Alma-Ata to the year 2000: reflections at the midpoint.* Geneva: WHO.

World Health Organisation. 1990. *The work of WHO 1988–1989 – biennial report of the Director-General.* Geneva: WHO.

2

Overview of primary health care in Southern Africa

KATHLEEN DENNILL

"There can be no human development without people being alive, healthy, knowledgeable and able to make a decent living." (UNDP, Human Development Report 1991)

CHAPTER OBJECTIVES

After reading this chapter, the student should be able to:

- discuss primary health care in the African situation
- explain how the Bamako and Accra initiatives have influenced primary health care in Africa
- discuss the role of the Organisation of African Unity in the development of primary health care in Africa
- discuss the development of primary health care in South Africa
- identify and discuss the strategies identified by the Department of Health in South Africa to implement primary health care
- discuss the vision for health in the new South Africa
- identify and discuss issues and trends in the new South Africa
- compare the primary health care programmes of the southern African countries.

2.1 INTRODUCTION

Many African countries acquired their independence about three decades ago and inherited health services that were based mainly in urban areas where most of the colonial inhabitants were settled. In the 1960s and the 1970s there was economic growth, which was accompanied by a modest expansion of health care, both geographically and technologically. However, since then, political instability and conflict in many areas, as well as a global economic recession, frequent droughts and the AIDS pandemic, have all had negative effects on the health status of Africans.

Any progress that had occurred in health development was curtailed and many countries are now faced with crisis situations and survival issues. Hospitals, health centres and equipment are in a state of disrepair and epidemics of preventable diseases are occurring and taking their toll, leaving a continent that has, to date, made very little progress in development and in the attainment of "health for all".

2.2 THE AFRICAN SITUATION

2.2.1 Indicators

Health and related socio-economic indicators put Africa among the least developed regions of the world. Examples of these include (UNICEF 1994:82–3):

- *Infant mortality rate* – 111 per 1 000 compared to 9 per 1 000 in industrialised countries
- *Life expectancy at birth* – 51 years compared to 76 years
- *Adult literacy rate* – 51% compared to 95%
- *Safe water supply* 43% compared to nearly 100%
- *Gross National Product (GNP)* – US $505 compared to US $18 884.

Various forms of aid have been poured into Africa to provide the required health care and to counter poverty, but have had very little long-term effect. More success has been attained in countries where a slow process of development, which has been initiated by the people themselves, has occurred.

In 1985 the Ministers of Health of the African region of the World Health Organisation committed themselves to use the primary health care approach to strengthen their national health systems. This resulted in a shift of emphasis to community-based health care. Since this commitment, the development of primary health care in Africa has been influenced by regional initiatives, which are discussed below.

2.2.2 The Bamako Initiative

In September 1987, when the economic situation in the region was deteriorating, the African Ministers of Health proposed a controversial plan to recover health care costs in sub-Saharan Africa. This plan was endorsed by the Organisation of African Unity in 1988. The objective of this initiative was to strengthen and improve health services as well as produce a health system that functioned adequately, especially at district and local levels. By instituting some form of cost recovery from the recipients of care, more services could be afforded and more people reached; equality of services being the objective.

A partnership between the community and the local health workers forms the basis of the process, with both management and financial control of the services as their joint responsibility. They therefore take control of their own health care and are able to channel resources where they decide they are needed most. Money is collected from the recipients of care and used for the enhancement of local services. This income could be used to cover the costs of drugs, stationery, fuel and even the salaries of supplementary health workers if required (Phillips 1990:271). This process would give "ownership of the health services" to the people of the community, the basis of a successful primary health care programme.

For this approach to succeed, however, financial and management support is necessary from central government (UNICEF 1994:64).

2.2.3 The Accra Initiative

This International Forum on Health was held in December 1991 in Accra, Ghana, to look at economic development and ways to break the cycle of poverty and inequality. The realisation that health is intrinsically linked to quality of life, formed the basis of the declaration and agenda for action that was drawn up. It was recognised that health care services alone would not result in a healthy nation. People in large parts of the developing world suffer persistent ill health, which is linked to extreme poverty and illiteracy. Development strategies must be implemented to improve this poor health environment by creating work opportunities and access to knowledge and skills. Only then will the health status of the community improve.

Developed countries, however, are not exempt from health problems. Excesses in lifestyles and overburdened environments produce vulnerable groups with health problems that must be addressed. In other words, the health of people is dependent to a large extent on a balance in a country's development strategy. To achieve this balance would require both developed and developing countries to share the knowledge gained through past experience and use it to avoid trading off health for economic gains.

The following is a summary of the proposals made in collaboration with the WHO and other international agencies to attain this (International Forum on Health 1991):

- Health-promoting activities could be identified and linked with income-generating activities and economic enterprise. These activities could then be made replicable on a global scale.

- An international health fund should be established, as well as a system of financial funding to link health objectives to economic enterprise, especially when vulnerable groups stand to benefit.
- Health criteria should be identified that would determine how resources are to be allocated. These could then be globally applied.

A task force was established to take these proposals further, in the hope that common solutions could be found to health problems by developed and developing countries acting together. Programmes could then be established that would be of use to help safeguard the health of people worldwide. These would be of special benefit to African countries, because they would help to ensure optimal care with available resources.

2.2.4 The Organisation of African Unity Summit

The Organisation of African Unity held a summit for heads of state and governments in July 1987. The result of this summit was a declaration on health as the foundation for development, which was produced in conjunction with the African regional office of the WHO. The declaration suggested that the governments of participating countries assess and define viable districts that could be managed by committees elected by the people. Each district would have its own budget and allow for decentralised community development, which would include community-based multi-sectoral health development activities. Support and resources would be required from the national government as well as international agencies such as the WHO and UNICEF. Self-reliance would be the basis of health development at district level (Monekosso 1989:53–6).

If primary health care is implemented in this comprehensive approach it should result in (Monekosso 1989:53–6):

- improved child survival
- less biological and economic wastage
- improved mental, physical and social fitness of the population, with considerable reduction in mortality and morbidity
- improved work productivity
- decreased disability in the population.

In November 1992 the International Conference on Assistance to African Children was convened. This was held at the request of the continent's leaders, to find ways to implement the goals for the survival, protection and development of children which were agreed to at the World Summit for Children held at the United Nations in New York in 1990. Africa's children account for only 10% of the world's child population, but one-third of the 40 00 children who die every day worldwide are African (OAU 1992:1).

FIGURE 2.1: Africa's children

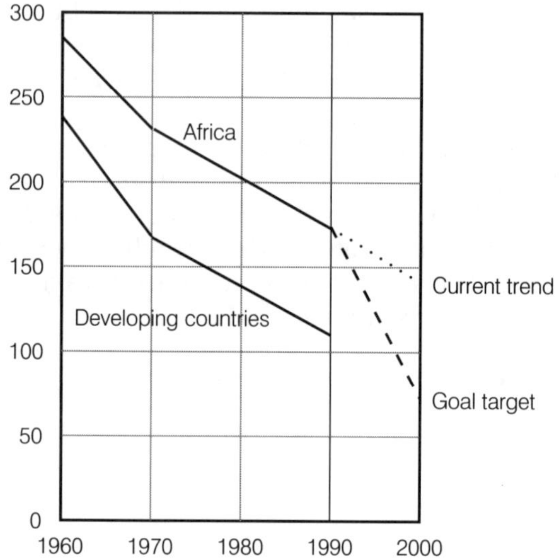

Under-five mortality declines: The under-five mortality rate (U5MR) has been halved since 1960, but an increased acceleration is needed if the year 2000 goal is to be achieved.

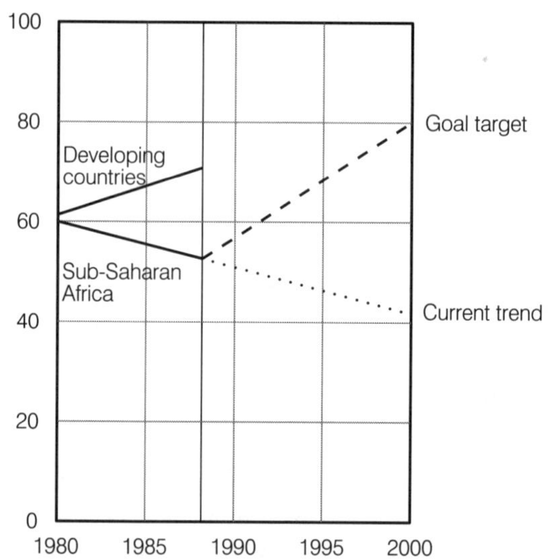

Basic education lost: While increasing in the 1970s in sub-Saharan Africa, the proportion of primary school entrance age children who reached grade 4 declined in the 1980s.

FIGURE 2.1: Africa's children *(continues)*

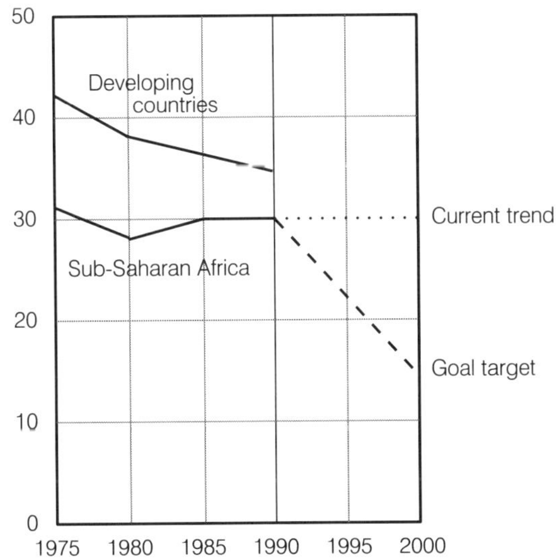

Nutrition progress stalled: Improvement of nutritional status in Africa during the 1970s stalled in the 1980s, while that for other developing countries improved.

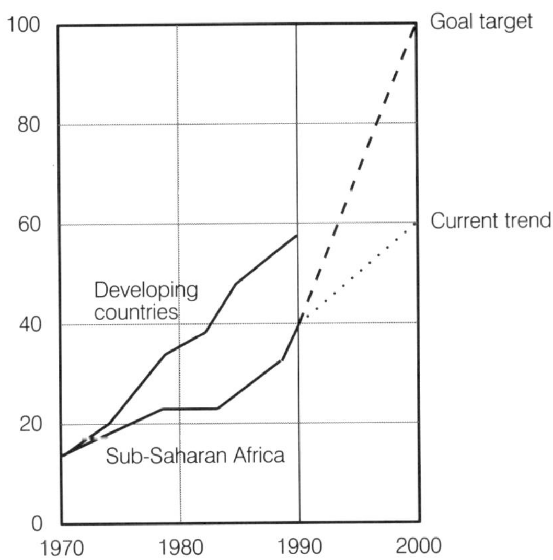

Gains in rural water: The proportion of the population with access to safe drinking water in rural areas has increased, but is still far from the goal of universal access by the year 2000.

Source: OAU (1992:17)

The goals of this summit were to provide basic health, nutrition, education and the necessary supporting services to children and to determine practical guidelines as to how these goals could be attained by joint African intergovernmental collaboration.

2.3 PRIMARY HEALTH CARE IN SOUTH AFRICA

2.3.1 The South African health system

The South African health system has evolved from different origins; the two main contributors being Western medicine and the various African cultures with their traditional tribal medicine. This has resulted in the development of two health systems in this country, alongside each other, with Western medicine having the official status.

The national health system as we know it has evolved in an unplanned and haphazard manner. It was influenced during the colonial period by both the British administration and the Boer republics. The health care system that developed out of these political changes was haphazard and the situation was further exacerbated by the discovery of diamonds and gold.

After the unification of South Africa in 1910, fragmentation of the health services occurred due to legislation that gave the four provinces control over their own health matters.

The Gluckman Commission of 1944 recognised this problem and called for a single, national health department that would serve "all sections of the population, according to their need, and without regard to race, colour, means or station in life" (Van Rensburg *et al.* 1992:61).

Unfortunately, the recommendations of this commission were never implemented and the apartheid era, after 1948, introduced legislation which enforced the segregation of health services and a separate development policy. The resultant homeland policy created nine more health departments to add to the five already established and this whole structure became very expensive and inefficient.

Health reform started in the 1970s with the economic recession. The result was a swing in the direction of self-reliance and privatisation, to try to reduce the financial burden on the state. To complicate the situation, there was escalating political and labour unrest. Against this background the *Health Act*, No.63 of 1977 was promulgated. It was an attempt to bring about fundamental reform in South African health care. It clearly defined the duties, the powers and responsibilities of the respective health authorities. Encouragement was given to the private sector to participate in supplying health care and a comprehensive approach was emphasised, with the preventive aspect taking a more prominent place. The aim was to assure reasonable access to health care for the entire population at community level (Van Rensburg *et al.* 1992:36–91).

In 1986 the government formulated a National Health Plan, with the objective of meeting the health needs of all the inhabitants of South Africa. This plan was based on the Alma-Ata principles of comprehensive primary health care and gave a firm political commitment to the implementation of such a service. The emphasis of the new endeavour would be on the prevention of disease and the promotion of health through community-centred services which advocate community participation and a multi-disciplinary approach. National strategies were identified with the idea that the future health delivery system would be developed as a unitary structure.

The emphasis on primary health care was taken a step further in 1989 when the National Health Policy Council accepted the following resolution: "The only way to provide an affordable health service to all the inhabitants of the Republic of South Africa, is by means of a partnership between the state and the private sector based on the National Health Services Plan, with the emphasis on primary health care." (Department of National Health and Population Development 1992:1)

The new direction that health care took in the 1980s was given statutory backing by the *National Policy for Health Act*, No.116 of 1990. It emphasised the following four principles:

- Individuals should take responsibility for their own and their families' physical, mental and social well-being.
- Costs incurred by individuals for health care should be recovered from them, but the indigent must be accommodated.
- The private sector should be encouraged to provide health services that are in the interest of the public.
- State and local authorities should provide a comprehensive health service that takes into consideration all available resources.

In May 1991 the government's intention to provide primary health care to all the people was made clear in the National Health Service Delivery Plan. It stated that during 1990–95 an affordable, comprehensive health service should be developed, which would be planned according to priorities identified by the communities themselves.

This plan recommended (Van Rensburg *et al.* 1992:81–88):

- reorganisation of health services to regional and local level, with the local authorities taking responsibility for most primary health care services
- that health services be democratised and community participation be advocated
- the right of admission of all population groups to public hospitals
- the introduction of community-orientated training of health personnel

- that the formula for health financing make available more funds for primary health care clinics.

2.3.2 Strategies for primary health care in South Africa

The Department of National Health and Population Development established a committee on primary health care to identify ways of implementing the 1986 National Health Plan. They produced a document, subsequently amended, to identify strategies or plans of action for implementing primary health care in South Africa. National strategies taking into consideration the political, social, economic and technical factors were developed.

The mission of the primary health care plan was . . . "to ensure the provision of cost effective primary health care to all the inhabitants of South Africa." (Department of National Health and Population Development 1992:6)

The 1992 edition of the document is discussed below, under each element or component of primary health care as identified by the WHO. The strategy for addressing each element was determined by the following process. Objectives were identified and to meet them, a plan of action and a process of implementation was decided on, with time constraints for each step. Methods of monitoring and evaluating progress were also established. The strategies determined were as follows:

- *To make information concerning the prevailing health problems and the methods of preventing and controlling them, available to the population.* Health education is a vital strategy of health care at all levels. To be accepted, health education must be culturally sensitive and suitable to the needs determined by each community. Health education should not be given by the health professionals alone; for it to be successful, a multidisciplinary, intersectoral approach must be used.

  In order to meet the requirements of the first component of primary health care, the following objectives were identified:
  - to network both national and international levels in order to facilitate the exchange of ideas and resources
  - to establish resource centres to provide and produce health education material and information about resources available elsewhere
  - to determine health education needs in the community
  - to initiate and facilitate the involvement of institutions and organisations in health promotion
  - to assist with the development of suitable learning resources, by supporting training in health education for health care workers
  - to ensure the effectiveness of health education towards achieving health for all

- to encourage an understanding and knowledge of "self" and its influence on perceptions of health, illness, disease and sickness.

- *To promote the provision of food and proper nutrition.* Adequate nutrition forms the basis of health; without it "health for all" is not attainable. This element, perhaps more than any other, has a reciprocal interaction with other elements. The success of one is determined by the other. A multidisciplinary and intersectoral approach is imperative to attain the objectives of this element. Two identified objectives were:
  - the promotion of the provision of foodstuffs. The following factors all have an impact on the provision of food and must be taken into account: the economic situation, employment levels, commodity prices and the performance of the agricultural sector. Food supplementation forms part of this strategy, and includes the provision of food to deprived groups or individuals to meet their minimum requirements when there is no other source available,
  - promotion of correct nutrition. Health education and training form the basis of any programme on nutrition. Facilities must be developed to train the personnel needed from the different disciplines to carry out these programmes.
- *To ensure an adequate supply of safe water and basic sanitation.* Safe water for drinking purposes should be colourless, odourless, pleasant to taste and free from disease-producing organisms and other agents. It should be available within walking distance and a minimum of 20 litres per person per day is required. Sanitation must be safe in that there should be an adequate number of toilets and an effective system of removal and disposal of household waste. There are no accurate statistics on the percentage of the population in South Africa that have access to safe water and adequate sanitation, but it is low. The objective is to ensure that by the year 2000, 70% of the South African population have access to the following services:
  - adequate safe water
  - effective toilet facilities
  - refuse removal systems
  - effective effluent disposal systems.
- *To ensure the provision of maternal and child health services,* including family planning (child spacing). Women and children constitute a major health care priority. The morbidity and mortality in this group are high and some of the causes can be prevented by simple, easily-implemented means. They constitute a large proportion of the population and, by promoting their health, the social and economic burdens on the community can be reduced. The objectives to attain these are to:
  - promote safe pregnancies

- promote safe contraception and provide counselling about child spacing and fertility, for all
- monitor growth and development of children
- promote school health services
- promote good nutrition and prevent malnutrition
- provide special services for children when required
- promote the development and training of personnel for mother and child health care.

- *To ensure immunisation against the major infectious diseases.* The immunisation of children is one of the most cost-effective means of improving child survival. The objectives of such a programme are to:
  - reduce morbidity and mortality by immunising children against the six preventable childhood diseases (measles, tetanus, tuberculosis, poliomyelitis, pertussis and diphtheria), as well as mumps and rubella
  - prevent the occurrence of neonatal tetanus and reduce the incidence of TB meningitis
  - create a management data information system.

- *To prevent and control local endemic diseases.* Endemic diseases can be divided into communicable and non-communicable diseases that include chronic diseases of lifestyle. Management of these conditions would be possible if the following objectives are met. They are to:
  - identify diseases that are endemic
  - manage, control and monitor endemic diseases in a specific area.

  The role of the epidemiologist is to identify the disease profile of the different areas within the country and to identify the important factors that influence these profiles. This information forms the basis on which the strategy of preventing and controlling diseases is planned. The following are important factors that can influence the disease profile in different areas:
  - age distribution
  - level of urbanisation
  - level of socio-economic development
  - state of the environment.

- *To appropriately treat common diseases and injuries.* To a large extent the success of the primary health care service and its credibility will depend on the successful management of these "minor ailments". Care given must be holistic, taking into consideration the context of the illness or condition and the environment in which the individual lives.

  The registered nurse, who is the health worker who fulfils this task in many primary health care services where there is no doctor, requires further training. However, most of the courses developed to meet this need

FIGURE 2.2: Infant mortality rate comparisons per 1 000 live births (1996)

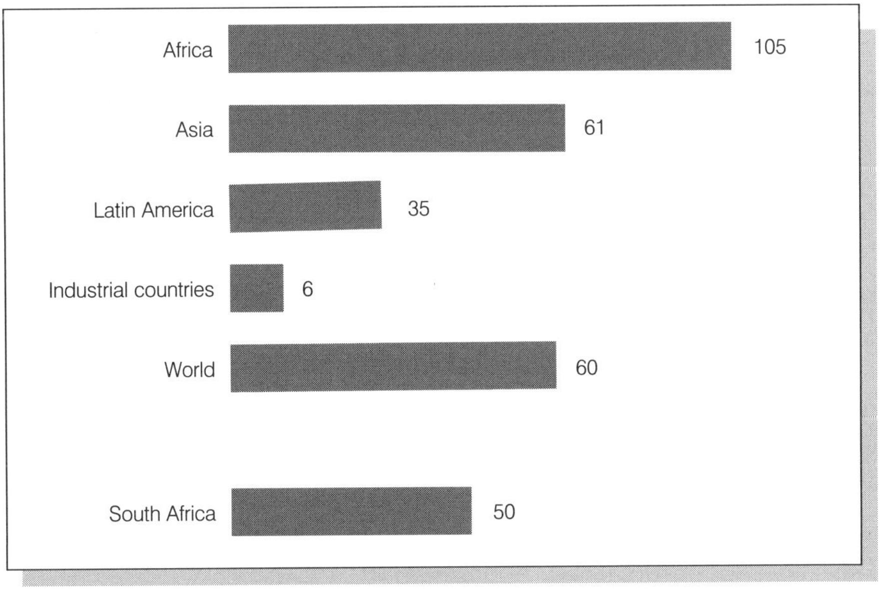

Source: UNICEF (1998:105–106)

FIGURE 2.3: Percentage contraceptive coverage (women of reproductive age)

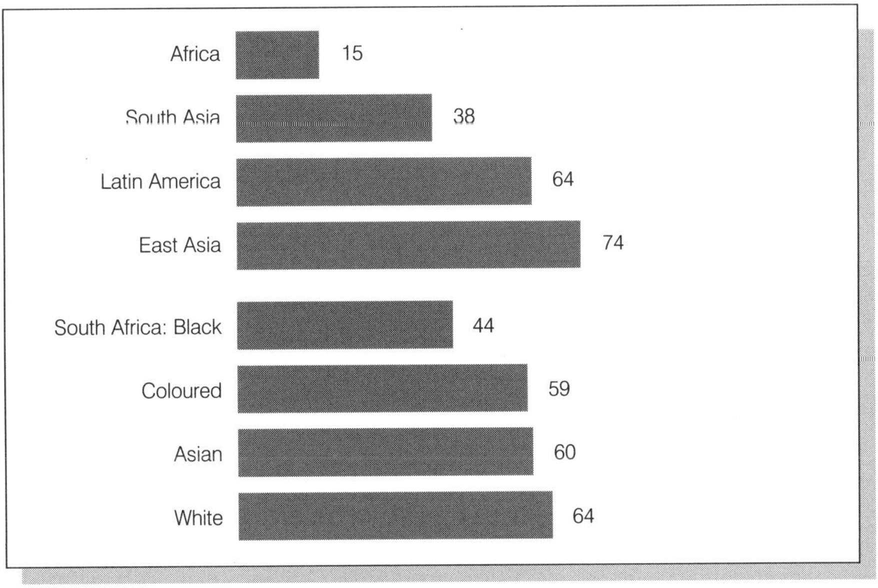

Source: UNICEF (1998:121) & Department of National Health and Population Development (1992:18)

FIGURE 2.4: Immunisation: percentage coverage of population under one year of age (1996)

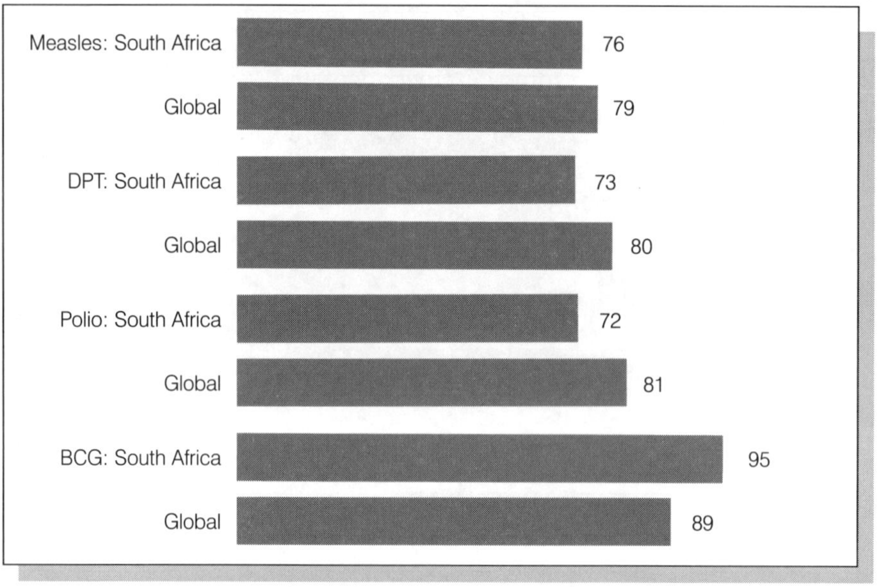

Source: UNICEF (1998:104–105)

FIGURE 2.5: Incidence of notifiable conditions per 100 000 population in South Africa (1992)

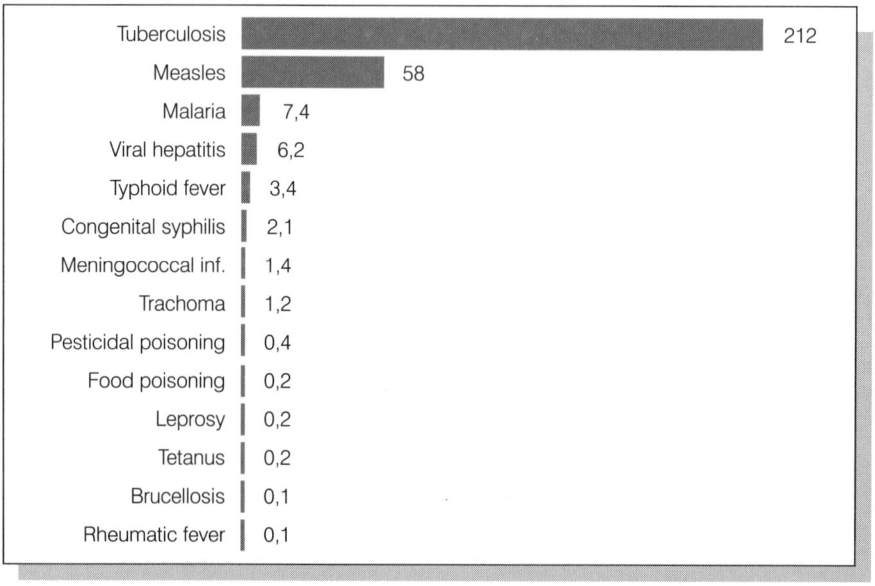

Source: Department of National Health and Population Development (1993:34)

emphasise the physical assessment, diagnosis and treatment of individuals, which is the curative aspect of the primary health care service, and neglect the communities' need for health care. This could result in primary health care workers becoming curative orientated, rather than preventive and promotive, and could result in the individual becoming the recipient of care and the community at large being relegated to a lesser position of importance, as it has in the past.

The objectives set out to meet this element of primary health care are to:

- educate and train health personnnel appropriately, efficiently and effectively, according to the available human resources
- develop systems that allow for continuity of care with efficient referral mechanisms and facilities
- deliver special care to high-risk groups
- develop cost-effective management protocols and efficient prognostic indicators.

- *To ensure the provision of essential medicine* (DNHPD 1992:1–63). A programme is required to meet the objective of providing essential, safe, effective and affordable medicines and vaccines to all who need them.

Progress was made towards attaining many of the objectives given above. However, the lack of information available, especially in rural areas, made the identification of community needs difficult and as a result, the planning of health services inefficient.

Training and education for health personnel was curative and hospital-based, rather than primary health care orientated and community-based. Another problem was and still is that much of the restrictive legislation of the apartheid era is still in place and will take years to unravel. This placed restrictions on the amount and on the speed of reform possible. The fragmented health service of the previous government, with its 14 departments of health, has been disbanded and realigned, but the process has proved to be difficult, which has complicated the implementation of reform.

Primary health care formed an important part of the previous South African health system. However, equality, affordability, acceptability, accessibility, availability, effectiveness and efficiency of health services all still require addressing if the goal of optimal health is to be attained for all South Africans. Yach *et al.* (1990:39) state, "The residual effects of apartheid on health will still need to be addressed and much effort will be required to develop a way of reducing existing race and social class inequities in access for and use of health care and health related services."

2.3.3 A vision for health in South Africa

The African National Congress's (ANC) final draft of its health plan was made available to the public in May 1994, at the time when the party came into power in South Africa, after winning the first democratic elections ever held. The health plan is based on the belief that every individual has the right to achieve optimal health. Aspects of the plan were clarified in the White Paper on Reconstruction and Development (RDP) which was published in September 1994.

The government is responsible for ensuring that health services are available to all South Africans and the ANC is committed to using the primary health care approach as the underlying philosophy to attain this restructuring of the health system. A National Health System was to be established under a single government structure to co-ordinate all aspects of health care in South Africa. This reconstruction would involve the complete transformation of the whole delivery system.

(a) Principles that form the basis of the health plan

The following are based on the proposals of the ANC (1994(a):19–20):

- *Equity.* Health for all cannot be acquired through the supply of equitable health services alone but rather through the achievement of equitable social and economic development. The need for employment, education, adequate housing, water, sanitation and electricity are all vital if "health for all" is to be attained.
- *Right to health.* This principle is based on the premise that each individual has the right to attain optimal health and the State must provide the environment in which this can be achieved.
- *Primary health care approach.* Comprehensive primary health care as identified by the WHO, forms the basis of this approach. It includes all aspects of community development and community involvement, which are imperative if the system is to be successful. Through this approach the inequalities in access to health services in rural and deprived communities will be a priority for improvement.
- *A single, comprehensive, equitable and integrated national health system must be created.* This system will be in control of all structures dealing with health, both public and private. It will be responsible to the people and all racial, tribal, ethnic and gender discrimination will be eradicated.
- *Co-ordination and decentralisation of services.* Clinics, health centres and independent practitioners will be the first contacts the people will have with the health system. Authority and control over the funding will be decentralised to the lowest level possible compatible with rational planning and the maintenance of good quality care.
- *Priorities.* The groups regarded as being the most vulnerable, such as mothers and children, the disabled, the underserved in rural areas and

those with debilitating diseases and conditions such as AIDS, tuberculosis, gastro-enteritis, heart disease and trauma, will be given priority care.

- *Promotion of health.* Attention must be given by health workers to the importance of health education, especially with regard to sexuality, child spacing, oral health, substance abuse, environmental health, occupational health and healthy lifestyles. Traditional healers and alternative health care practitioners must be integrated into the team of health workers.
- *Respect for all.* A charter of patient's rights will be introduced to ensure the right of all people to be treated with dignity and respect.
- *A health information system.* There is a need for appropriate and reliable data, which is essential for good planning and management. This will improve the efficiency of the service.
- *Additional components of primary health care.* To cover the specific needs of primary health care in South Africa, the new government added more components to the eight of the WHO. They are emergency, occupational and mental health services. To further support the programme, priority is to be given to the development of a national health information system and a research programme is to be established that will link research with health policy and practice (ANC 1994(b):44–50).

(b) The National Health System

The main reason for the health department's existence is to ensure access for everyone to good-quality health care. To achieve this the government must:

- create, monitor and change when necessary, the framework or system in which health is promoted and health care is delivered.
- be a major provider of services.

The changes planned for the health services in 1994 were primary health care based, and aimed to decentralise services with the emphasis being placed on community care. The aim was to decentralise management and introduce district health systems. For decentralised health care to work, central co-ordination is required "within an integrated, unique and comprehensive national health service" (ANC 1994(a):59). The structure planned allows for a continuum of health care with a referral system that should permit an easy, logical movement between primary, secondary and tertiary services within one co-ordinated system. To achieve this goal, a multidisciplinary health team approach to health care is necessary, which must include both public and private providers, as well as adequate input from support services such as laboratory services and pharmaceutical suppliers.

FIGURE 2.6: The relative importance of different functions at different levels of the health system

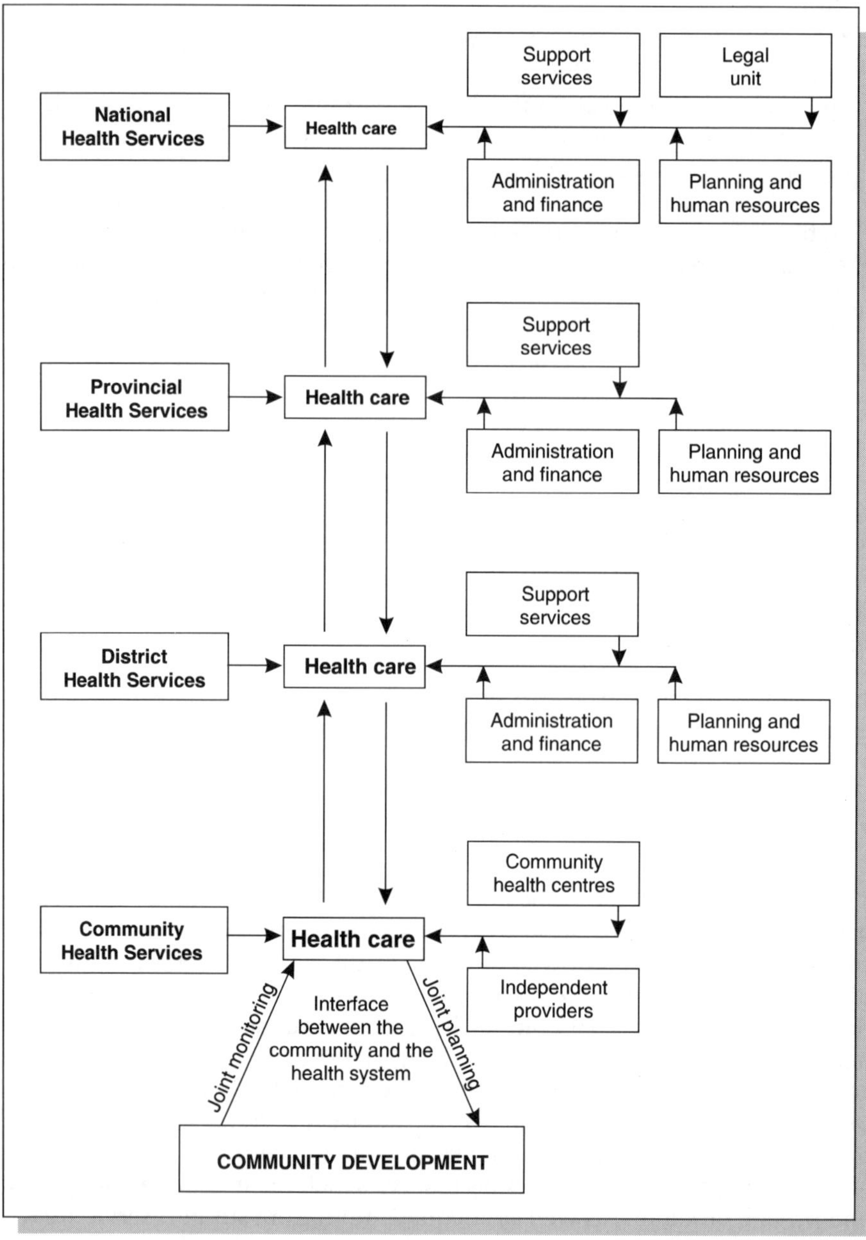

Source: ANC (1994(a):60)

(1) *National level*

At central government level there will be a single National Department of Health. This department will be led by the Minister of Health, who is advised by the Intersectoral National Development Committee, which consists of the ministers of all the sectors of government that have an impact on health, e.g. water, agriculture and housing.

The National Health Authority is the body which, under the direction of the Minister of Health, is responsible for the provision, development and co-ordination of all health care in South Africa. The National Health Authority allocates the health budget and is responsible for health policy and legislation. This body is advised by the National Health Advisory Body, which consists of representatives of the statutory bodies and members of the national associations of health professionals, non-government organisations, trade unions and national community organisations. This department is responsible for the co-ordination of both public and private health care and for international liaison.

Academic hospitals are accountable to the National Health Authority, but will enjoy a fair amount of autonomy and will be encouraged to generate their own funds where possible. They are an important part of the national resource, forming a vital part of the health referral system as well as offering facilities for research and human resource development and training. These institutions have commanded a large proportion of the health budget and rationalisation is likely to make funds available to primary health care services.

(2) *Provincial level*

At this second tier of government there are nine provinces, each with their own provincial legislature. Each provincial health authority is responsible for all aspects of health care required by the people of that province. This includes emergency care, hospital care, environmental safety and a suitable referral system. They are also responsible for the support, monitoring and evaluation of services given at district level.

The department at provincial level will be run by the Provincial Director of Health Services, who is responsible to the Member of the Executive Committee for Health, who is elected to the provincial legislature. The main function of the members of the Executive Committee is to identify needs within the province and allocate resources accordingly.

The management committee, which comprises the Provincial Director of Health Services and the directors and heads of provincial departments, is responsible for the day-to-day running of the service. Included in this is the control of specialist hospitals. However, management of these institutions will be largely the responsibility of those in charge of each hospital.

FIGURE 2.7: Proposed organogram of the NHS at the national level

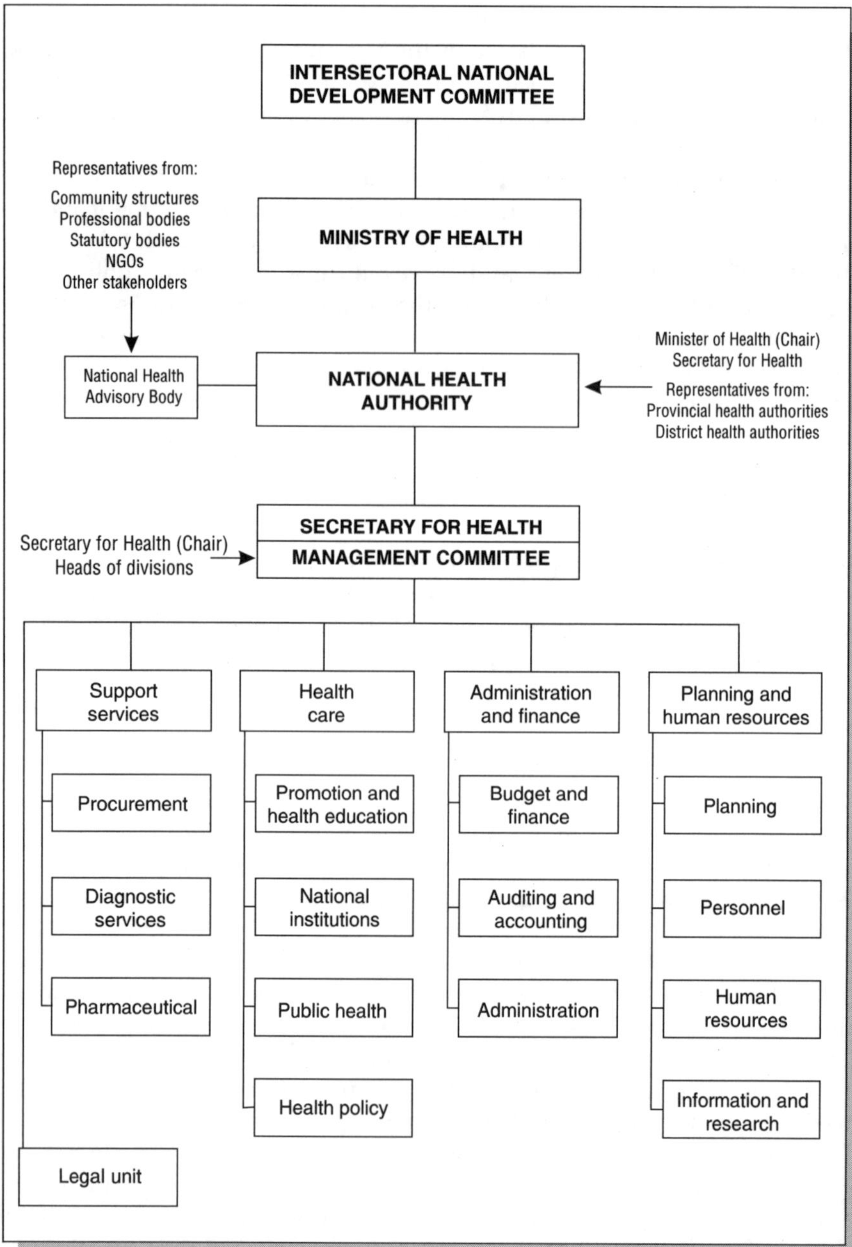

Source: ANC (1994(a):69)

To facilitate community participation, a Provincial Health Advisory Authority will be established and will consist of representatives from professional bodies, health worker organisations, trade unions and community organisations as well as members from the private health sector.

FIGURE 2.8: Proposed organogram of the NHS at provincial level

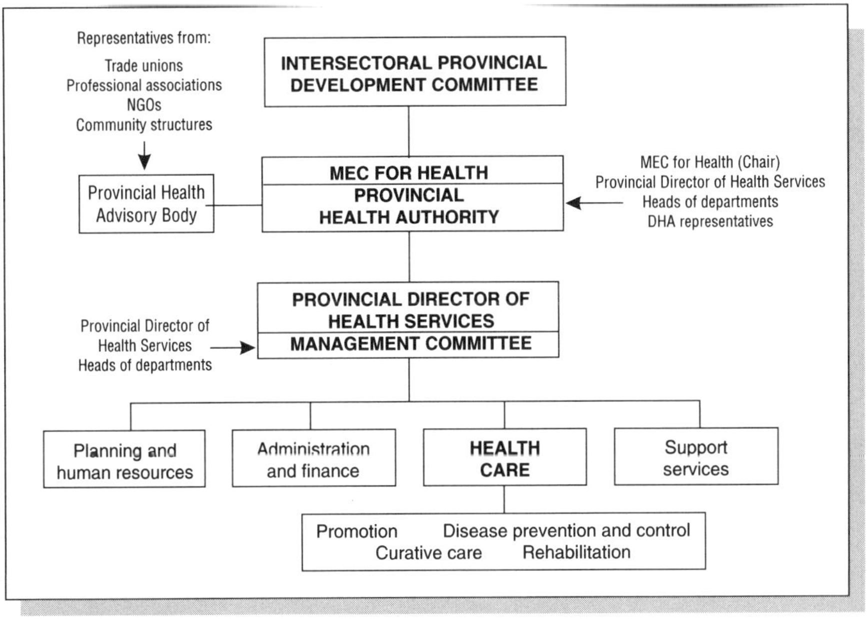

Source: ANC (1994(a).65)

(3) District level

Each province will be divided into districts according to functional and geographical determinants. The size of each district will be determined by the population, and will vary from 200 000 to 750 000, depending on the density of the population between rural and urban areas. To realign health services in this manner makes sense, since it allows for a more equitable distribution of resources. However, it will threaten some of the existing local authorities, because boundaries will change and two or three local authorities will be incorporated into one district.

The district health authorities will be accountable to the elected political authorities, and all community health services, private and public, will be their responsibility. The authority will comprise representatives from the local authorities and the community health authorities, and should also include some of the service providers from the district clinics, health centres and community hospitals.

Advising the district health authorities is the Intersectoral District Development Committee, which consists of members from any other sector which influences health, e.g. education, water affairs and industry. The District Health Advisory Body allows for community participation at district health level. This body is made up of representatives of the community health committees, community-based organisations, trade unions, professional bodies and health worker organisations.

FIGURE 2.9: Proposed organogram of the NHS at district level

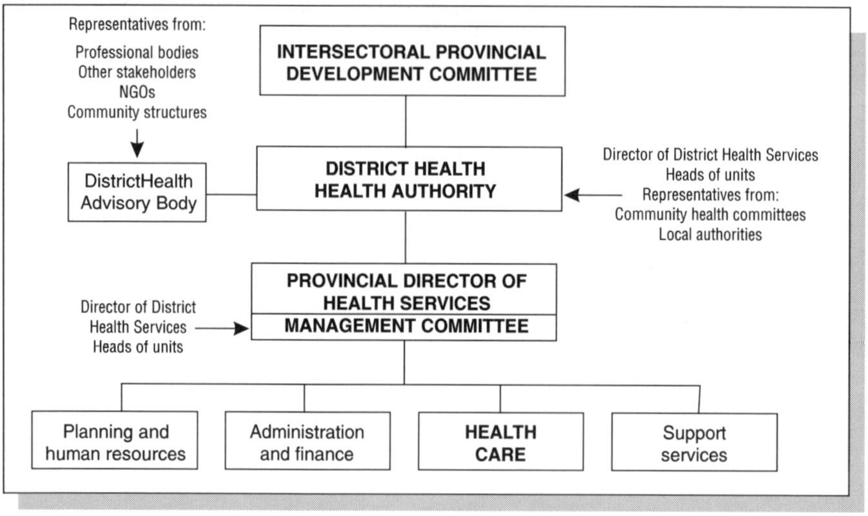

Source: ANC (1994(a):63)

The most important function of the district health authorities will be to provide primary health care services to all members of the community. These authorities will receive and allocate the budget to supply these services. Services will include clinics, community health centres, community hospitals and emergency services. In the first phase of the Reconstruction and Development Programme (RDP), a model or pilot health district is being developed in each province, which can be replicated.

As part of the district health service, at the interface of community-based health care with the basic health services at ground or village level, community participation is vital to the success of primary health care. The importance of this level of care is emphasised in the new health plan and the RDP.

(4) Community level

Each community living in a geographical area served by community health services will be encouraged to form an intersectoral community development committee. This committee will advise and work in co-ordination with the community health committee on all development projects as well as the use of resources in the area.

FIGURE 2.10: Proposed organogram of the NHS at community level

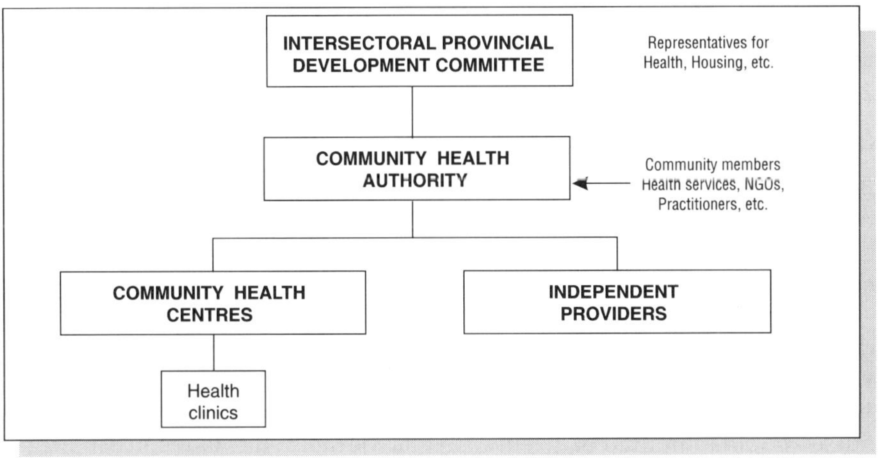

Source: ANC (1994(a):61)

The Community Health Committee will consist of elected community members who will serve on a voluntary basis. Representatives will be drawn from the health services, non-government organisations and health practitioners in the area. They will liaise with those employed to run all the community health services and especially the community health centre of each district. They will help to prioritise health needs and determine local health policy. The community health centre in each district forms the heart of the district health services and provides preventive, promotive, curative and rehabilitative care.

Clinics will provide similar services at a less specialised level. All permanent clinics should have water, electricity and some method of communication. Some areas are to be serviced by mobile clinics (ANC 1994(a):61–70).

Important projects initiated by the RDP as part of socio-economic development and which could impact positively on health, are:

- a primary school nutrition scheme
- rural water provision

- a national literacy programme
- small-scale farmer development
- free health care for under-sixes and mothers, pre- and postnatal, at state facilities
- clinic building
- an AIDS awareness and prevention campaign
- urban renewal projects.

2.4 PRIMARY HEALTH CARE IN OTHER SOUTHERN AFRICAN COUNTRIES

2.4.1 Botswana

(a) Current situation

Botswana gained its independence in 1966. It is a landlocked country with two-thirds of the land consisting of the Kalahari desert. The eastern region of the country is more fertile and habitable and is the most populated. The north-west corner consists of an extensive swamp, the Okavango Delta.

The population was 1,5 million in 1996, with an annual population growth rate of 3,1%. The life expectancy rate is 52, the infant mortality rate 40 per 1 000 and the gross national product (GNP) per capita is US $3 020 (UNICEF 1998:94–107). In 1985 there was a doctor : population ratio of 1:7 000 and a nurse : population ratio of 1:700, with a favourable shift to the urban areas.

Since independence the country has been transformed and the per capita GNP has risen five times. The reason for this has been the emergence of a mineral sector in the economy, which had been centred on beef production prior to independence. Poverty, however, is still a problem because the formal sector still only employs approximately 20% of the population. The rest of the population depends on subsistence farming and other non-formal activities for an income.

(b) Health policy and strategies

When Botswana gained its independence it inherited a health service that was predominantly curative and urban-based. Primary health care was adopted as the main strategy for health care, using a comprehensive approach so that community development is addressed. The National Development Plan VI (1986–1991) of the Botswana government gives the highest priority to productive employment creation and rural development, the objective of the plan being to break the cycle of poverty which is still a major problem. This, in turn, would result in the inhabitants of Botswana attaining a minimum living standard that is consistent with health. The

Ministry of Health is responsible for the health of the nation and is assisted by the private sector, which consists mainly of mining companies and Christian missions. Also at central level is the Rural Development Council which co-ordinates the District Development Committees, which are brought together annually to discuss important issues relating to development. At village level there are further community committees, which involve the community members in their own health care and development.

Health services in Botswana include health posts, clinics, health centres, district hospitals and referral hospitals. The country is divided into districts which are administered by a District Council. Health at this level is the responsibility of the district health team, which offers operational support to the clinics and health posts. The team is multidisciplinary and consists of a public health physician, a community health nurse, a health inspector, a tuberculosis officer, a nutrition/health education officer, a rehabilitation social welfare officer and support staff (WHO 1987:80).

(c) Effectiveness

Botswana has made remarkable strides since independence. Its human development is the best in sub-Saharan Africa. Health services have been developed and 89% of the population now has access to health services, with 85% living within a 15 km radius of a facility (Macgregor 1991:147). However, the effects of poverty are still prevalent, with many children still suffering from undernutrition, resulting in a lowered resistance to infections. Immunisation coverage is nearly 80%, while accessibility to safe water is 93% and to adequate sanitation 55% (UNICEF 1998:102).

2.4.2 Lesotho

(a) Current situation

The Kingdom of Lesotho is an independent (1966) developing nation and is the only country in the world with all its land more than 1 000 m above sea level. It is completely surrounded by the Republic of South Africa, on whom it is reliant for a large proportion of its GNP, which is provided by Lesotho citizens who work on South African mines. Most of the mountainous regions are not accessible by road and can only be reached by small aircraft or on horseback.

The population of Lesotho was 2 million in 1996, with an annual population growth rate of 2,6%. The life expectancy rate is 58, the infant mortality rate 96 per 1 000 and the GNP per capita is US $580 (UNICEF 1998:94–107). There are approximately 114 medical doctors, who practise mainly in urban areas, and 900 practising nurses (Gary and Warren 1991:11).

(b) Health policy and strategies

The government of Lesotho officially accepted the primary health strategy of Alma-Ata in 1979 and has set about implementing it in three five-year plans. The country is divided into 18 districts (health service areas), which can operate independently and which have a three-tier referral system. The private sector and non-government organisations are responsible for about 50% of health care. Policy is determined and health development monitored at national level. At district level the communities are given responsibility for their own health and health development and elect their own committees. These committees are established by law which was promulgated in 1981. Membership usually includes traditional leaders and healers.

Since resources are limited, priority is given to providing new services to rural areas which have previously received little or no service. In other areas, established services have been upgraded when possible.

Major endemic diseases in Lesotho are tuberculosis, sexually-transmitted diseases and typhoid. About 20% of all children under five are considered to be underweight (WHO 1987:143–5).

(c) Effectiveness

Primary health care programmes are considered a success in Lesotho, in that they have been initiated and implemented by the Basotho people themselves and are community orientated. However, the inaccessibility of the mountainous areas and the wide distribution of people in these areas, make the satisfactory distribution of services almost an impossibility. This has resulted in many rural people still being underserved.

Only 62% of the people have access to safe water and 38% access to adequate sanitation (UNICEF 1998:103). Projects to improve both of these have been implemented over the last decade and the situation is gradually improving. Immunisation coverage is also improving slowly, with approximately 60% of children being fully immunised in 1992 (UNICEF 1994:68). The environmental problems need to be addressed by multisectoral efforts, since at present too much is left to the health sector alone.

2.4.3 Namibia

(a) Current situation

Namibia is a vast country on the western side of southern Africa, where a large proportion of the land is desert. It was known as South West Africa before independence in 1990 and was administered by the South African government. The population was 1,6 million in 1996, with only 34% of these people living in urban areas. The others are sparsely distributed over the rest of the country. The annual population growth rate is 2,7%, and the life expectancy at birth is 56 years. The infant mortality rate is dropping and was 60 per 1 000 in 1996. The GNP per capita is one of the better ones in Africa, at US $2 000(UNICEF 1998:94-107). The mainstay of its economy is its mineral resources and agriculture.

Prior to independence, services were fragmented along racial lines in a similar way to South Africa, which resulted in the establishment of 11 different health administrations. These health departments were supported by church missions, which supplied a large proportion of the services in the north of the country. As in South Africa, this complex situation resulted in inequality of services and focused largely on the curative aspect of health care.

(b) Health policy and strategies

The Ministry of Health and Social Welfare adopted the primary health care approach after independence. Major restructuring within the health service was necessary. To implement this, the Directorate of Primary Health Care was established, appropriate policies were developed and the necessary legislation was promulgated. The emphasis of the health services moved from curative to preventive and promotive care.

The new health service is headed by the Department of Health and Social Welfare at central level. At regional level the country was divided into a much more manageable four regions. These regions are responsible for supervising and monitoring the district services. Each district comprises at least one district hospital with its associated health care centres, clinics and other services. The use of mobile clinics is important because of the remoteness of rural villages and the large areas that are sparsely populated.

(c) Effectiveness

There is no doubt that the new health service has been successful, and health statistics bear this out. There are, however, constraints that limit the Namibian Health Service's success in implementing primary health care for all. They are:

- vast distances for some to reach facilities
- lack of public transport and inaccessibility of some areas
- lack of education
- a sparsely distributed population.

Intersectoral collaboration is working in Namibia, with all sectors that have a part to play being involved in planning and implementing programmes. The result is the optimal use of available resources to the benefit of the people (Ministry of Health and Social Services 1992:1–81).

2.4.4 Zimbabwe

(a) Current situation

Zimbabwe is a landlocked country to the north of South Africa. Most of the developed infrastructure is found on the plateau or "highveld", which runs diagonally across the country from south-west to north-east. When the country gained its independence in 1980 it inherited a health system which was inappropriate and unequally distributed. The bulk of the government's spending on health had been on curative care in urban areas. The health care situation had also been negatively affected by the armed struggle, especially during the last few years before independence. The services had been badly disrupted and more than half of the clinics did not function. Many of the mission hospitals which served the rural areas had had to close during this period.

The population of Zimbabwe in 1996 was 11,5 million, with an annual growth rate of 3,0%. The life expectancy rate is 49 and the infant mortality rate 49 per 1 000. The GNP per capita is US $540(UNICEF 1988:94–107).

(b) Health policy and strategies

The inherited health services were fragmented and fell under five different authorities; the Ministry of Health, local authorities, church missions, industry-based clinics and private clinics (Macgregor 1991:148–9). There was also a high concentration of services and personnel in urban areas, with rural areas often being underserviced.

In the years after independence the government attempted to redress these inequalities. In 1982 the government published its policy document "Planning for equity in health care", which advocated a primary health care approach. It aimed to provide access to health services that would be made more comprehensive and integrated. The underlying causes of ill health, such as poor living conditions, inadequate nutrition and lack of safe water, were to be addressed.

Programmes were introduced to give free health care to those earning a limited income. A national immunisation programme was implemented, diarrhoeal control programmes were introduced and the supply of essential drugs was improved. Hospitals, health centres and clinics were built or rebuilt and by 1989, 771 more clinics were functioning than before independence. Money spent by the state on health care was increased, along with social benefits like the setting of minimum wages, food subsidies, expanded education and water development.

(c) Effectiveness

Zimbabwe's achievements in health were impressive in the 1980s and allowed many people access to health care services for the first time. The impact on the health of people was, however, limited because of the prevailing poverty. Financial problems placed constraints on further development of health care. As a result, many of the old problems are still present. Health planning remains centralised and there is a serious shortage of staff at all levels.

2.4.5 Other

There are two other countries in the southern African region that should be mentioned. They are Angola and Mozambique, both of which were brought to their knees by the armed conflict within their borders. Both are listed among the 10 least developed countries of the world. Mozambique is of special importance to South Africa, since a steady stream of refugees constantly crossed the border into South Africa during the civil war. This placed further demands on the resources available for our own communities and thus affected the health status of our own people.

2.5 FUTURE PROSPECTS FOR CO-OPERATION ON HEALTH MATTERS

There have been only limited, mostly informal, links between South Africa and other countries of the region because of the past political situation and the conflict in the area. For successful reconstruction to occur, links should be created that are of equal benefit to both South Africa and her neighbours. Areas where collaboration would be of value include (Beattie *et al.* 1993:930–2):

- control and eradication of infectious diseases
- development of a disaster relief and surveillance system
- development of a regional drug policy
- managing of human resources, their training and flow within the region
- strengthening the health research capacity of the region
- use of grants and funds, available to the area, to the benefit of all the role-players.

These links can occur through informal networking between professionals or academics or more formal links between governments. The co-operation should encourage collective action and allow the region to confront various difficult health matters in a constructive way.

2.6 SUMMARY

For primary health care to be successful in South Africa, it needs "to be rescued from the political arena of political sloganeering, but it is not an easy task" (Coovadia 1994:9). It must be entrusted to the people, since this form of health care is dependent on community participation and promotes self-reliance and self-determination. Some question the success of community participation, because it is a time-consuming, slow and uncertain process, and would rather emphasise the provision of preventive, promotive, curative and rehabilitative services at community level. However, to meet the challenges in primary health care in the future, we must study and learn from the past. Primary health care is an ongoing process which must develop over time and change to meet new situations. It is the only feasible means of meeting the health needs and improving the situation of the people of southern Africa.

Bibliography

African National Congress. 1994(a). *A national health plan for South Africa.* Maseru: Bühr Mapping and Printing.

African National Congress. 1994(b). *The reconstruction and development programme.* Cape Town: ABC Printers.

Beattie, A., Rispel, L. and Booysen, M. 1993. Problems and prospects for health sector links in the southern African region: the role of South Africa. *Social science medicine.* Vol. 37, No. 7:927.

Benetar, S.R. 1990. A unitary health service for South Africa. *South African Medical Journal.* Vol. 77:441.

Bierman, J. 1994. Legal limitations in primary health care practice in South Africa. *International journal of medicine and law.* Vol. 13, No. 1:141–53.

Coovadia, J. 1994. Forsaking the revolution. *University of Natal: Focus.* Autumn Edition:9.

Department of National Health and Population Development. 1992. *Strategy for primary health care in South Africa.* Pretoria: Government Printer.

Gary, F. and Warren, J.K. (Eds) 1991. *Primary health care in the Kingdom of Lesotho.* Battle Creek: W.K. Kellogg Foundation.

International forum on health. 1991. Accra initiative on health: declaration and agenda for action. *International nursing review.* 1992, Vol. 39, No. 2:46.

Jinabhani, C. 1993. High costs of poverty. *University of Natal: Focus.* Autumn Edition:5.

Kelly, J. 1990. *Finding a cure: the politics of health in South Africa.* Johannesburg: South African Institute of Race Relations.

Lobstein, T. (Ed.) 1984. *Namibia: reclaiming the people's health.* Nottingham: Russell Press.

Macgregor, J. 1991. Towards human-centred development: primary health care in Africa. *Africa Insight.* Vol. 21, No. 3:147.

Ministry of Health and Social Services. 1992. *The official national primary health care: community-based health care guidelines.* Namibia: Ministry of Health and Social Services.

Monekosso, G.L. 1989. *Accelerating the achievement of health for all Africans: the three-phase health development scenario.* Brazzaville: WHO.

Organisation of African Unity and United Nations Children's Fund. 1992. *Africa's children, Africa's future: human investment priorities for the 1990s.* Addis Ababa: OAU.

Owen, C.P. (Ed.) 1988. *Towards a national health service: proceedings of the 1987 NANDA annual conference.* Cape Town: NAMDA Publishers.

Phillips, D.R. 1990. *Health and health care in the Third World.* Hong Kong: Longman.

Steyn, H.J. 1990. A strategy for primary health care – towards health for all. *Journal of comprehensive health.* Vol. 1, No. 2:130–2.

Streefland, P. and Chabot, J. 1990. *Implementing primary health care.* Amsterdam: KIT Publications.

United Nations Children's Fund. 1994. *The state of the world's children.* Wallingford: Oxford University Press.

United Nations Children's Fund. 1998. *The state of the world's children: 1988.* New York: Oxford University Press.

Van Rensburg, H.C.J., Fourie, A. and Pretorius, E. 1992. *Health care in South Africa.* Pretoria: Academica.

White Paper. 1994. *Reconstruction and development programme.* Cape Town: CTP Book Printers.

World Health Organisation. 1987. *Evaluation of the strategy for health for all by the year 2000: seventh report on the world health situation.* Brazzaville: WHO.

Yach, D., Pick, W. and Padayachee, N. Critical issues for community health in South Africa in the 1990s. *Journal of comprehensive health* Vol. 1, No. 1:38–49.

3

The multidisciplinary public health team

LAETITIA KING

"Coming together is a beginning, keeping together is progress, and working together as a team is success." (Lightfoot 1991:1)

CHAPTER OBJECTIVES

After reading this chapter, the student should be able to:

- discuss the concepts which appear in this chapter
- develop an understanding of the multidisciplinary nature of public health
- discuss the nature of a multidisciplinary health team
- list the members of a multidisciplinary, intersectoral health team
- form an opinion of the value of teamwork and of a multidisciplinary, intersectoral approach to health care provision
- discuss the concept "leadership" as a requirement for effective teamwork
- evaluate the role of the nurse as a member of the multidisciplinary health team.

3.1 INTRODUCTION

The following statement, by participants attending the 1978 World Health Organisation conference at Alma-Ata, sets the scene for a multidisciplinary, intersectoral team approach in health care delivery:

> "The Conference strongly reaffirms that health, which is a state of complete physical, mental and social well-being, and not merely the absence of disease or infirmity, is a fundamental human right and that the attainment of the highest possible level of health is a most important worldwide social goal whose realization requires action of many other social and economic sectors in addition to the health sector."

The ultimate goal of all health care workers should be to help the public attain an optimal level of health and so realise this fundamental human right. It must, however, be accepted that this goal will not be possible without the active participation and co-operation of all members of the multidisciplinary health team, a team that must include all individuals who can contribute in some way to the well-being of the community.

Only when a holistic approach to health care is adopted - an approach which necessitates a multidisciplinary and intersectoral co-operative team effort - will it be possible to effectively address the health care needs of all individuals and groups in the community.

The outcome will be influenced by the level of involvement of all the individuals who form part of the particular health team. The success of public health outcomes depends on teamwork, as does the outcome of any other health-related activity. In all instances, success depends on the effective contribution and co-operation of every member of the team.

3.2 THE MULTIDISCIPLINARY NATURE OF PUBLIC HEALTH

In order to understand the multidisciplinary nature of the health team, it is necessary to clarify what is meant by the concept "public health".

The definition of public health, suggested by Winslow as far back as 1920, is still widely accepted today (Bury and Svensson 1994:8):

> "Public health is the science and art of preventing disease, prolonging life, and promoting physical health and efficiency through organized community efforts for the sanitation of the environment, the control of community infections, the education of the individual in principles of personal hygiene, the organization of medical and nursing service for the early diagnosis and preventive treatment of disease, and the development of the social machinery that will ensure to every individual in the community a standard of living adequate for the maintenance of health."

The current debate about public health was brought about, *inter alia,* as a result of a need to restructure and reform health care systems, following increasing public awareness of health as an important social goal. Central to this approach should be the objective of placing public health "not at the periphery of medicine but at the centre of health" (Bury and Svensson 1994:9). These authors suggest the following criteria must be inherent in any definition of public health:

- public health is population-based
- it advocates a global and social model of health
- it requires an intersectoral and multidisciplinary approach
- it emphasises a systems approach to health management, to harness the organised efforts of society to promote health and population empowerment.

Last, as cited by IJsselmuiden (1993:57), explains the multidisciplinary and intersectoral nature of public health by stating that it is a "combination of sciences, skills, and beliefs that are directed to the maintenance and improvement of the health of all the people through collective or social actions".

IJsselmuiden (1993:67) maintains that, since public health is essentially multidisciplinary and intersectoral in nature, it is "not the property of a specific profession, nor of professionals in general, but both as a practice and a social movement it belongs to all".

Public health can thus be described as a discipline which includes the many activities performed by all individuals or groups involved in any aspect of health care, in an attempt to assist the community with the prevention or reduction of disease occurrence, and by so doing to increase the health and well-being of the population as a whole.

3.3 CO-ORDINATED MULTIDISCIPLINARY AND INTERSECTORAL ACTION TO ACHIEVE HEALTH GOALS

Before discussing the principle of a co-ordinated multidisciplinary and intersectoral approach to health care provision, it is necessary to be familiar with the meanings of a few of the key concepts. A discussion of the concept "multidisciplinary team" is included further on in this chapter. In the 1992 publication, *Strategy for Primary Health Care in South Africa,* the concepts "intersectoral action" and "co-ordination within the health sector" were defined as follows:

- *Intersectoral action:* action in which the health sector and other relevant sectors collaborate on the achievement of a common goal, the contributions of the different sectors being closely co-ordinated
- *Co-ordination within the health sector:* this concept implies organised collaboration as necessary among those providing the services at the same and different levels of the health system, in order to make the most efficient use of resources, as well as within the various categories of health workers following agreement on the division of labour (Department of National Health and Population Development 1992:65–6).

A multidisciplinary and intersectoral approach is not only a way of satisfying individual health needs, but is also the most effective way in which the many pressing health issues facing the world should be addressed. Collaboration and co-operation between those whose actions influence the health and well-being of the community must take place not only at local level, but should extend to country, regional and international levels.

The need to promote multidisciplinary, intersectoral co-operation is widely supported. The International Conference on Primary Health Care at

Alma-Ata recognised intersectoral co-operation as one of the guiding principles for achieving health goals, and stressed that "the improvement of health required more than the services delivered by the health sector alone" (WHO 1986:13). Particular reference was made to the vital role played by other sectors, such as agriculture, animal husbandry, food, industry, education, housing, public works and communications, in improving the health and well-being of the community. The Strategy for Primary Health Care in South Africa, as developed by the Department of National Health and Population Development in 1992, echoes this view and maintains that "the team approach in the rendering of primary health care is of fundamental importance to ensure its success" (Department of National Health and Population Development 1992:8).

Dr Nakajima, the WHO Director-General, in reaffirming the commitment of the WHO to multidimensional involvement in health care provision in his address to the WHO Executive Board on 17 January 1994 said: "The new health partnership we want to achieve stresses the interdependence of all sectors, communities and individuals, and the need to share resources and responsibilities in a spirit of respect and solidarity." (WHO 1994:1). Dr Nakajima continued by referring to the multidimensional nature of health, and said that synergy and intersectoral co-operation are vital to the achievement of health as a part of economic and social development (WHO 1994:16).

The ANC policy guidelines on health, adopted at a national conference on 28 to 31 May 1992, include the following statement regarding intersectoral co-operation (*SA medical journal* 1992:393):

> "At all levels of government the health services should promote intersectoral co-operation to promote the health of communities. The health service will play a role in co-ordinating government authorities responsible for sanitation, water supply, food and agriculture, housing, and other social services. To the extent that a threat to public health is identified, the health service will ensure that the necessary steps are taken to remove such a threat."

3.4 EFFECTIVE MULTIDISCIPLINARY TEAMWORK, INTERDISCIPLINARY CO-OPERATION AND INTERSECTORAL COLLABORATION

To achieve successful intersectoral action in health care provision, a truly multidisciplinary health team must be available. Teamwork, which must be seen as a process rather than an end in itself, is defined by the WHO as co-ordinated action, carried out by two or more individuals jointly, concurrently or sequentially. According to the definition, the following prerequisites are vital for effective teamwork (WHO 1988:6):

- common, agreed-on goals

- a clear awareness of, and respect for, others' roles and functions on the part of each member of the team
- adequate human and material resources
- supportive co-operative relationships and mutual trust
- effective leadership
- open, honest and sensitive communications
- provision for evaluation.

3.4.1 The advantages of effective teamwork

The effectiveness of a multidisciplinary health team can be described as the success it has in addressing the total health care needs of the community, and by so doing improving the health and well-being of the community. To achieve such success, the team must be innovative, creative and flexible, and must have clearly defined and shared objectives to cope with the constant changes which occur in the environment and the social system. In addition, the members making up such a team must provide the right combination of expertise and experience to achieve effective results.

Poulton and West (1993:921) are of the opinion that if a team is to be effective, it must possess a definite vision and shared objectives, it must practise participation and sharing of information, it must commit itself to excellence and must have strong support for innovation and the initiation of new ideas.

The advantages of effective teamwork are many and varied. Pritchard (1981:47) refers to the value of teamwork with regard to increasing job satisfaction, reinforcing health education, improving the standards of care and making the best use of the special skills of team members. What is, however, of greatest value to the recipients of health care is the synergistic effect of successful teamwork and interdisciplinary co-operation. Effective teamwork addresses the critical need for closer co-operation between all elements of the health team, a factor which is of vital importance if the ever-increasing health care needs of a changing society are to be addressed effectively. There is "no stronger force in this world than a group of people working willingly toward the same specific goal" (Lightfoot 1991:1). Without the synergism achieved through effective teamwork, optimal health for all members of the community will never be attained.

In discussing the value of sharing in a multidisciplinary team approach to community assessment, Dreyer *et al.* (1993:117) refer to various advantages which also apply to teamwork in general. These include:

- the sharing of knowledge and information to the benefit of the community
- the sharing of the unique talents of team members to enhance the outlook of the individual members

- the delegation of functions and responsibilities to appropriate team members according to their expertise, knowledge and experience
- the meaningful interpretation of collected data about the community.

3.4.2 Leadership as a requirement for effective teamwork

For any team to function effectively, there must be effective leadership. The community health nurse, because of her unique position in the community and at the different levels of the health system, is often in the position where she is required to assume a leadership role, and consequently plays a major role in facilitating change and development in the community. The leadership skills required to do so effectively, are seen as crucial for the successful outcome of the projects and programmes planned for a particular area. The success of the leader will depend on the person's ability to develop the required skills, as well as on his or her understanding of the dynamics that affect the leadership process. It should, however, be noted that, whether the leader of the public health team happens to be a physician, a nurse or any other member of the team, is not important. What is important is that, as a member of a multidisciplinary team dedicated to ensuring the best possible health care for the community, the leader should, firstly, be able to recognise the areas of need that should be attended to, and secondly, be able to make the best possible use of the members of the team to ensure that the identified needs of the community are attended to effectively. Leadership doesn't have to be grandiose or high-powered, but to be able to lead the multidisciplinary health team with success, its leader needs to have a vision and commitment, and would definitely benefit by undergoing professional training in the art of leadership. According to Roemer (1988:443), public health leadership "requires generalists who can appreciate the enormous variety of problems affecting the health of populations and the very wide range of strategies necessary to promote health and prevent disease, or to facilitate treatment when prevention has failed". These generalists are not necessarily physicians, but should be team members who have a thorough understanding of the concept of public health, and who should be well prepared to fulfil the responsibility of leadership so urgently needed.

There are various leaderships styles which the leader might apply. These include the following:

(a) Autocratic leadership

Leadership styles with a high degree of control are described as autocratic, authoritarian, bureaucratic or paternalistic. A modification of this style of leadership, in which the leader retains control but permits some input in decision-making, has been described as that of the mature autocrat or diplomat.

Using an autocratic style of leadership, the leader would:

- give step-by-step guidelines
- be directive, tell people what to do and rely heavily on detailed policies, procedures and protocols, as well as strict control and feedback mechanisms
- provide feedback in the form of praise and recognition for a job well done or give constructive criticism
- be more task-orientated, in that the leader must ensure that the job is completed.

In practice, it is often found that the leader decides on a more autocratic leadership style when working with a group who have little knowledge, experience or skills, or lack confidence in their ability to achieve a specific task. For example, it is highly probable that detailed instructions, job descriptions and close supervision and control would be needed when working with newly qualified, inexperienced health care workers. Once the group has matured and gained more confidence, the leadership style could probably move along the continuum to a more relational or people-orientated approach, in which group participation in decision-making could be encouraged and less detailed direction and control would be needed.

(b) Democratic leadership

Leadership styles that promote greater autonomy in the working situation and which are more relational or people-orientated, are described as democratic, participative and egalitarian. Collaborative and collegial leadership styles are extensions of the purely democratic leadership style and can be used to facilitate increasing self-leadership and autonomy in the work situation as the maturity level of the worker rises. This leadership style is crucial in terms of the Reconstruction and Development Plan and the National Health System of South Africa, in which groups are encouraged to become self-sufficient and self-supporting.

The leader who uses a more democratic style of leadership will be more inclined to consider the group's or individual members' needs and feelings, and would also be more successful in developing good interpersonal relationships and encouraging information-sharing between the various team members.

In this style of leadership, the leader needs to:

- explain the need for decisions to be taken and provide opportunities for clarification

- sell his or her ideas, vision and goals
- share ideas and facilitate decision-making by giving the necessary support and guidance.

To do this, the leader needs to encourage participation in the planning and decision-making process, delegate responsibility and accountability for implementing tasks to an increasing extent as the maturity level of the group grows, and develop a mutual trust relationship between group members over a period of time.

The democratic leadership style, with variations, is probably the one most frequently used in the community health field. It is certainly the style most appropriate when working with the health team, community leaders and experienced workers in the field.

(c) Laissez-faire or permissive leadership

The laissez-faire leadership style is also referred to as a free-rein or a permissive leadership style. This means that the leader takes little or no responsibility for the work done or for the individuals or groups involved. Only if requested to do so, does the leader participate and act in an advising, guiding, counselling capacity (Bernhard and Walsh 1990:58).

When deciding on the best leadership style to adopt, the leader will be able to influence to a large extent the success with which the health needs of the community will be met. In order to do so, the leader needs to:

- determine the knowledge, skill and competency level of the individuals or groups with whom she or he will be working
- decide with the group which duties and responsibilities can be safely delegated
- draw up detailed plans with the group or individuals concerned as to how the tasks will be delegated and implemented
- decide with the group who will be responsible and accountable for the jobs to be completed
- ensure with the group the development of appropriate control and feedback mechanisms that are effective and acceptable in terms of local needs.

3.4.3 How can effective teamwork and interdisciplinary co-operation be promoted?

Constructive working relationships must be developed to ensure co-operation and negotiation between team members, and to allow knowledge and experience to be shared.

To ensure that the community will benefit from co-operative team efforts, it is necessary to look beyond the level of academic or professional expertise of a fellow team member, and to consider the overall value of the contribution made to the welfare of the community. Not only will such an attitude contribute greatly to the fostering of mutual respect, trust and co-operation among the various members of the team, but the synergistic results achieved will be of tremendous benefit to the well-being of the community.

If effective teamwork and team cohesion are to be initiated and maintained, all members of the team need to critically assess their individual roles in order to identify areas of possible interdependence with other categories of workers. This will require role clarification by the various members, as well as a willingness to share responsibilities with others.

3.4.4 Intersectoral collaboration and equity in health

According to the WHO (1986:123), equity forms the "unifying theme of a policy for intersectoral action for health". One of the recommendations put forward during the 1986 Technical Discussions of the 39th World Health Assembly, states that WHO member states should "take action to ensure that national strategies for health for all are developed and implemented as an integral part of an equity-orientated development strategy" (WHO 1986:127). In planning and decision-making, the health sector should collaborate with other sectors when formulating and implementing appropriate health care strategies.

All people in the community have a right to be healthy, and should therefore have equal access to health care. If equity in health is to be achieved, a multidisciplinary, intersectoral approach to health care provision must be followed. A single individual or discipline will never be able to supply the community with all the care needed to ensure the achievement of optimal health. Nor will the efforts of the health sector alone be sufficient to enable the community to achieve equity in health. The members of the multi-disciplinary health team will have to accept that only once there is extensive collaboration, will it be possible to provide the community with the best possible solutions to identified health care needs and problems.

3.4.5 Barriers to teamwork and a multidisciplinary approach to health care delivery

There are various barriers that could adversely affect teamwork and a multidisciplinary approach to health care delivery. These barriers should be avoided or overcome at all costs if the community is to benefit from the combined input of the multidisciplinary health team.

(a) Barriers related to official policy and the nature of health care services

Factors such as fragmentation of health care services, inadequate referral systems, the inequitable distribution of health personnel, the approach to health strategy development and general resistance to change in the health industry, may adversely affect teamwork and interdisciplinary co-operation.

In spite of efforts by the WHO and its member states to increase intersectoral involvement in the development of health policies, it notes that in many instances the development of health strategies is controlled mainly by the health sector, with the emphasis on a curative approach, and inadequate attention is paid to intersectoral collaboration. Although intersectoral co-operation is not promoted as a panacea for all health problems, we are reminded by the WHO (1986:13) of the tremendous contribution it can make towards improving socio-economic and other conditions that adversely affect the health and well-being of the community.

Reluctance to recognise the many changes taking place in society and in the health care industry will negatively affect intersectoral co-operation and teamwork. In order to ensure effective teamwork, change must be accepted as a means towards better health care services. Moji (1990:124) maintains that "the organisational survival of the health care industry, looking at the nature of its mission in the society, is not a matter of choice or being efficient but of being adaptive". Adaptation, or change, is not always easy, and is perceived by many people as a threat to their security. Resistance to change in health care provision not only affects the health care services, but ultimately adversely affects the community which depends on the health care provided. Reluctance to change therefore not only inhibits the improvement of health services, but is tantamount to negligence and borders on the unethical.

With regard to the distribution and utilisation of health personnel, Pick (1992:301) maintains:

> "In spite of the poor coverage of the population by professional health workers, not much provision has been made for non-professional (and often more appropriate) types of health worker. The exclusive use of professional health workers is not only expensive, but also ensures that they retain control over the provision of health care."

Such an approach does not improve interdisciplinary relationships, and ultimately deprives the community of much-needed health care.

The following clearly describes the lack of teamwork that is evident, not only in primary health care, but in many areas of multidisciplinary health care provision (Poulton and West 1993:920):

> "Multidisciplinary working, particularly within primary health teams, is also difficult. Separate lines of control, different payment systems leading to suspicion about motives, diverse objectives, professional barriers and perceived inequalities in status, all play a part in limiting the potential of multiprofessional, multi-agency teamwork. These undercurrents often lead to rigidity within teams,

> with members adhering to narrow definitions of their roles, preventing the creative and flexible responses required to meet a variety of human needs presented. They are also likely to lower morale. For those working under such circumstances efficient teamwork remains an elusive ideal."

A multidisciplinary, intersectoral approach to the planning and provision of health care is fundamental to the successful implementation of any health care system. If the health care system is to address the needs of the population effectively, it is necessary to acknowledge that all members of the multidisciplinary health team, including the individuals, families and community groups, fulfil a vital role in the health team.

(b) Barriers related to the attitudes of health workers and of the community

Factors such as professionalism, professional jealousy and status prevent many team members from co-operating with each other to the benefit of improved health care provision. "Problems of professional co-operation can be traced back through the history of each professional group's separate development" (Poulton and West 1993:919). The same authors also discuss the Harding Committee findings regarding difficulties in co-ordinating primary health care teamwork in the United Kingdom, and refer to the following prerequisites suggested by the committee for successful team integration:

- a common team objective which is accepted and understood by all members
- a clear understanding by each team member of his or her role, function and responsibilities
- a clear understanding by each team member of the role, function, skills and responsibilities of the other team members
- mutual respect for the role and skills of each team member, allied to a flexible approach.

Successful teamwork requires a concerted effort by all team members to accept each other and to recognise the contribution made by each member. Schein, as cited by Chell (1985:110), recognises the potential problems that could arise in a group should status factors interfere with the group objectives, and warns that "just bringing a group of people into interaction does not ensure a good working group". A change in attitude towards other members of the team is necessary if effective teamwork is to become a reality.

Public ignorance also adds to the poor relationship that exists between certain sectors of the health team and the community. Van Rensburg *et al.* (1992:295) refer specifically to public ignorance and prejudice that exist about the role of supplementary health care workers in South African health care, but add that in some instances the established health professions are also guilty of not acknowledging the important contribution that these members of the team could make to the provision of comprehensive health care services.

(c) Barriers related to the training of health workers

Training of professional health care workers in public health is largely compartmentalised and very rarely integrated. According to IJsselmuiden (1993:68), this makes the current training of members of the health care team inappropriate for a multidisciplinary approach to health care.

An integrated, multidisciplinary and intersectoral approach to health care must be promoted by providing training facilities that are available to all whose work impacts on the health of the community. The WHO (1988:5) refers to multiprofessional education, orientated to the priority health needs of the community, as being in line with the policy of the World Health Organisation to "foster a type of educational programme for health personnel that will enable them to respond to the needs of the populations they serve as part of efforts to achieve the goal of health for all through primary health care".

Yach *et al.* (1990:38) maintain that an appreciation for the value of teamwork and the importance of multidisciplinary and intersectoral co-operation must already be initiated at the most basic student level. The training of all members of the health team must place a greater emphasis on the multidisciplinary team concept, and on the need for closer and more meaningful co-operation between all members of the health team. The following statement, put forward by a WHO Study Group on the team approach in health personnel education (WHO 1988:39), indicates that the study group supports the view of Yach *et al.*:

> "To sum up, experience indicates that, for best effect, formal multiprofessional education needs to be introduced early in basic or undergraduate educational programmes, continued throughout a curriculum, and then continued in post-basic, postgraduate and continuing education programmes."

There are, however, various constraints that have to be faced in the development of a curriculum that promotes multidisciplinary training. Whereas students are generally receptive to such an approach, Miller (1995:10) reports that "... faculty members clearly provide the greatest point of resistance, with academic turfism being a recurring theme". In addition, the warning is raised by Miller that the introduction of a multidisciplinary approach into a curriculum could be "... a logistic nightmare to schedule students and various health professionals to work together in community settings''. It is also mentioned by Miller that perceived financial disincentives could influence the willingness of institutions to adopt a multidisciplinary approach to the training of health care professionals.

3.5 THE MULTIDISCIPLINARY HEALTH TEAM

Cooney (1994:178) defines the term multidisciplinary as the ''... juxtaposition of various disciplines, sometimes with no apparent connection between them, for example chemistry, sociology and architecture'', and adds that, where members from such disciplines would work together as a team, they do not necessarily spend all their time working together but at times would ''... rely on themselves and on other members to achieve the goals or functions of the team''.

To appreciate the significance of a multidisciplinary team approach to health care provision, it is necessary to take note of the WHO definition in which a health team is described as ''a group of people who share a common health goal and common objectives, determined by community needs, to the achievement of which each member of the team contributes, in accordance with his or her competence and skill, and in co-ordination with the functions of others'' (WHO 1988:6). The WHO also maintains that since the nature of such co-operation will vary from society to society, and has to be determined according to relevant local needs and resources, no universally applicable composition of the health team can be prescribed.

Lock *et al.* (1992:92) refer to a team as a group of people who make different contributions towards the achievement of a common goal. In health care the common goal should be ''optimal health for all'', and should be the main objective of all members of the multidisciplinary health care team.

A multidisciplinary health team can be defined as a team whose members represent the widest possible spectrum of individuals and organisations concerned with, or involved in, any aspect that has a bearing on the health and welfare of the community, in an attempt to provide effective, comprehensive health care that will assist in the achievement of optimal health for all people.

3.5.1 The health team in a group context

Bobbitt *et al.* (in Chell 1985:107) define a group as ''a collection of individuals amongst whom a set of interdependent relationships exist''. Such interrelatedness should also exist between the various members of the health team. When Schein's interpretation of the formal functions of a group, as referred to by Chell (1985:108), is considered, the similarity between the following functions of groups, and the activities performed by the multidisciplinary health team, can be noted:

- groups work on complex interdependent tasks which are too difficult for any one member to perform
- a group acts as a means of generating new ideas or creating solutions
- groups fulfil a liaising and co-ordinating function
- groups assist in solving problems
- groups facilitate the implementation of complex decisions.

All these characteristics of a group should be evident in the actions of an effective multidisciplinary health team.

3.5.2 The need to expand the multidisciplinary health team

As a community develops, health care needs and the means of satisfying such needs, change. New dimensions of health care provision evolve, bringing with them new members to be included in the multidisciplinary team. This refers not only to new areas of specialisation in modern medicine and its support services, but also to well-established traditional health care providers, who previously were not acknowledged as part of the health team. Human resources are the most valuable assets that any country can possess, and available expertise should not be ignored if the highest possible level of health is to become a reality for all. The provision of holistic health care will only be successful if the health team is multidisciplinary in the widest possible sense

Glatthaar (1990:2) reminds us that a team committed to providing the best possible health care appropriate to the needs and priorities of the community should not permit itself the indulgence of exclusivity. If optimal health for all is to be achieved, it is necessary to develop a truly multidisciplinary health team that will transcend the traditional barriers between lay and professional people, and between professionals active in the various sectors of society that have an influence on community living.

A change in attitude on the part of all involved in health care provision is, however, necessary. There must, for instance, be closer co-operation between the providers of modern medicine and those involved in supplying traditional medicine. In this context Van Rensburg *et al.* (1992:340) suggest that the establishment of a new syncretic type of health care system in South Africa could be achieved by means of either coexistence, with traditional and modern medicine complementing each other as two independent sectors of health care, respecting the unique character of each other, or by integration of traditional medicine into the existing official medical care system. Whatever the approach is to be, closer co-operation between the different elements of health care provision is inevitable in a changing South Africa. Such development will require tolerance and an acceptance of the need for co-operation and mutual referral between traditional and modern medical care providers.

The community must be accepted as a full partner of the multidisciplinary health team. Members of the health team must be able to liaise and co-operate with individuals and representative committees in the community. The approach to health care provision adopted by the South African Department of Health emphasises in this regard the participation of the community, as well as the importance of strengthening community services and developing a district health system.

In order to appreciate the relevant importance of health care at the district level, it is necessary to take note of the way in which the concept "community" is interpreted in the National Health Plan (ANC 1994:61): i.e. it is used to "represent those people living in the geographical area served by a community health centre". It is envisaged that comprehensive primary health care will be delivered to the community through these community health centres (CHCs), and all members of the health team should therefore be knowledgeable about the composition and functions of the proposed community health centre teams. According to the National Health Plan, "the CHC team will include a full range of health workers in order to deliver a comprehensive service" (ANC 1994:61). The community will be represented on a community health committee by voluntary, elected community representatives, who, together with representatives from the health services in the area, NGOs working in the community, local health practitioners and others, will ensure that health priorities, as identified by the community, are attended to. The need to expand the multidisciplinary health team is therefore of paramount importance to ensure the successful implementation of an equitable health service in South Africa.

3.5.3 Composition of the multidisciplinary health team

To appreciate the significance of a truly multidisciplinary health team, it is important to remember that health is a complex, multidimensional concept which is inextricably linked with all aspects of daily living. If the health care needs of the community are to be addressed effectively, attention must be given to all the components that interact in making up a society, such as biological, physical, personal, social, legal, economic and political aspects. It is also necessary to consider how the various components influence health and health care services, and how, in turn, the availability of the health care services, or lack of them, affect various aspects of daily living.

Although the structure of the multidisciplinary team may vary according to the needs and locality of the community and the available resources, membership should not be limited to workers directly involved in health care provision or to those whose work has a direct influence on the improvement and maintenance of the health and well-being of the community. The team should also include individuals whose work may have an indirect impact on public health, such as those in the agricultural, religious, financial, educational and architectural fields. In addition, the team should also include the ordinary individual in the community – be it the patient and his or her family, or any other concerned individual or group who can assist the community to improve its health status.

The question as to who should be included in a multidisciplinary team that will supply holistic health care to all who may need it, can quite simply be answered as everybody who can in any way contribute to the health and well-being of the community. In this regard, Figure 3.1 provides a graphic representation of the multidisciplinary health team as suggested by Glatthaar.

FIGURE 3.1 The multidisciplinary health team

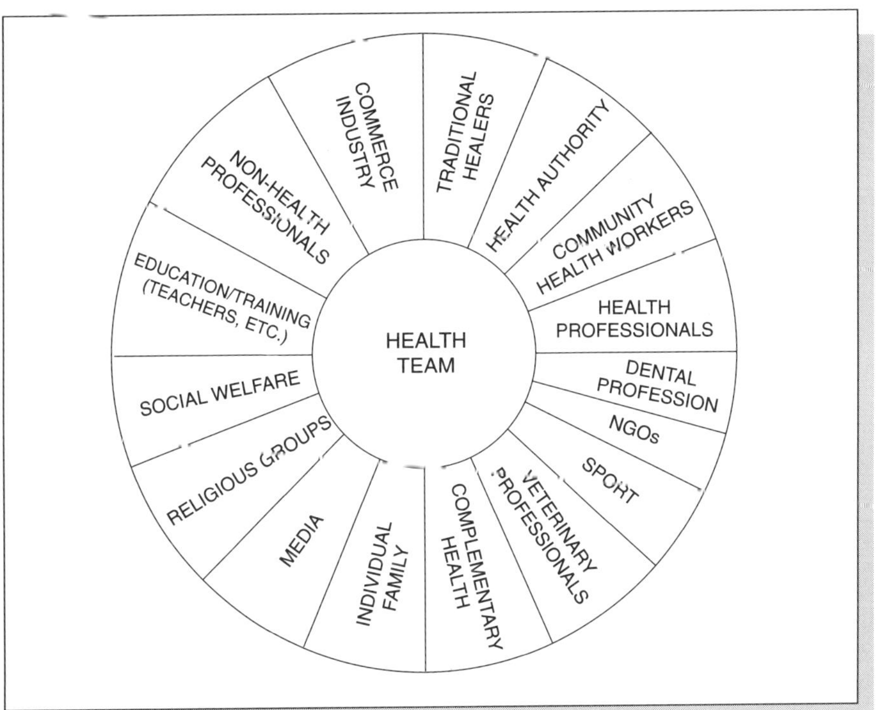

Source: Glatthaar (1990:2)

Van Rensburg *et al.* (1992) outline the personnel responsible for supplying health care in South Africa, and refer to two main categories of health care providers: those involved in the provision of official health care and those providing non-official health care. Stanhope and Lancaster (1992:28) divide health care providers into three groups: independent practitioners, dependent practitioners and support staff. In both these examples, the emphasis is on the direct provision of health care, without attention being given to the many disciplines that could have an indirect effect on the health and well-being of the community in a broader context.

Based on the premise that a health system, as an integral part of society, must be multidisciplinary and intersectoral, the following classification of members of the health team is suggested.

3.5.4 Classification of members of the multidisciplinary health team

Category A: Individual team members directly involved in health care provision

1. *Professionals in the health sector providing official health care: physicians, nurses, dentists, pharmacists, supplementary health care providers*
   The important role played in the hospital health team by supplementary health care providers such as the speech therapist, the physiotherapist, the radiographer, the social worker and the dietician, to mention but a few, is well known. In the community health field it is an accepted fact that professionals such as the environmental officer and the social worker form an invaluable link in the health team. The list of supplementary health care workers is extensive and the value of their contribution is immense.

   The following are the major categories of workers in supplementary health occupations in South Africa (Van Rensburg *et al.* 1992:294): audiologists; audiometrists; dental therapists; dieticians; electro-encephalographic technicians; food inspectors; health inspectors; masseurs; medical physicists; medical technicians; medical technologists; occupational therapists; optical dispensers; optometrists; oral hygienists; orthopaedic orthoptists and prosthetists; orthoptists; physiotherapists; podiatrists; psychologists; psycho-technicians; radiographers; remedial gymnasts; speech therapists.

2. *Individuals providing non-official health care: alternative health care professionals, traditional health care providers and lay care providers.*

Please note that the team members referred to by Van Rensburg *et al.* (1992) as providers of non-official health care enjoy varying degrees of recognition in the South African health care system.

(a) Alternative health care professionals

Subsection 1 (categories registered by the South African Council for the Associated Health Service Professions)

- homeopaths
- chiropractors
- naturopaths
- osteopaths
- certain herbalists.

Subsection 2 (groups of practitioners currently not registered under any Act of Parliament)

- reflexologists
- aromatherapists
- acupuncturists.

(b) Traditional health care providers

These include:

- diviners
- certain herbalists
- faith healers and prophets.

Traditional health care workers feature prominently in the provision of health care in South Africa. Large sectors of the South African population have in the past made extensive use of traditional healers in their quest for optimal health, and will continue to do so in the future.

(c) Providers of lay care

Lay care refers to health care which is provided by non-official and unskilled health care workers, and includes both an individual and a collective form, which Van Rensburg *et al.* (1992:309) refer to as self-care and mantle care. Self-care includes a variety of methods used by the individual to satisfy personal needs, such as those related to accommodation, clothing, nutrition and hygiene. It also refers to the responsibility of the individual to avoid harmful practices such as smoking and alcohol abuse. Mantle care includes care provided to each other by members of a particular small community. In this type of care, the providers and recipients know each other on a personal level, and also interact in a variety of social situations.

Specific mention must also be made of the various community-based health workers who are from, and selected by, the community. This category includes health educators, rehabilitators, traditional birth attendants and so forth.

Category B: Individual team members from sectors other than the health sector, involved indirectly in health care provision

It is in this area that the need for an intersectoral approach to health care becomes most meaningful. According to the WHO (1986:16), the sectors which, in addition to the health sector, have a major impact on health include: agriculture, nutrition, education, culture, information, environment, water, sanitation and industry.

The following list of professionals, whose work impacts indirectly on the health of the community, is not an exhaustive one, but merely attempts to illustrate the diversity of the team: agriculturalists; anthropologists; architects; demographers; economists; educationalists; engineers; environmentalists; industrialists; information science specialists; journalists; lawyers; politicians; religious leaders; sociologists; statisticians; town planners; veterinarians; welfare workers.

In addition to the team members listed in categories A and B, there are many individuals and organisations involved both directly and indirectly in health care provision. These include governmental health and related agencies, non-governmental and civic organisations, community support groups, trade unions, voluntary organisations and the private sector. All individuals, groups and organisations must work together as a team, for only through effective teamwork can the goal of optimal health for all be achieved.

3.5.5 The nurse as a member of the multidisciplinary health team

To appreciate the role of the nurse as a member of the multidisciplinary health team, brief reference must be made to the concept "community health nursing", in order to recognise how it forms part of the broader multidisciplinary concept of public health.

Hanlon, as quoted by Clark (1984:32), defines community health nursing as "a field of specialisation within both professional nursing and the broad area of organised public health practice" and maintains that it utilises the philosophy, content and methods of public health as well as the knowledge and skills of professional nursing. Lock *et al.* (1992:10) agree that community health nursing science is a specialised area of nursing, and stress that the community health nurse, when dealing with groups, families and individuals, must co-operate with the rest of the multidisciplinary team in order to achieve success. For a more in-depth discussion of the concept of community health nursing, see chapter 1 of Dreyer *et al.* (1993).

The vital role that the community health nurse plays with regard to achieving optimal health for the community is widely acknowledged. The importance of fulfilling this role within the multidisciplinary team concept, which is a vital characteristic of public health, needs to be emphasised.

It is important to note that membership of a team doesn't automatically ensure acceptance and recognition by the other team members. Acceptance of the nurse depends not only on her own professional abilities, or on the perceptions which other team members may have developed about her, but to a large extent on her own willingness to share responsibilities and involvement in health care provision with other members of the team.

The community health nurse is in an ideal position to assess the needs of the community, and to act as co-ordinator, facilitator, health care practitioner and referral agent within a team context, and in so doing, to ensure effective comprehensive health care for the community. Remember that, although the nurse plays a vital role in the provision of health care to the community, she is but one of a large number of contributors to the overall team effort. The nurse should therefore appreciate the importance of interdisciplinary and intersectoral co-operation, and to achieve success, must accept the team approach as the ideal way to solve the health problems of the community.

The community health nurse will have to be prepared to accept the many changes which are likely to occur in the health care system in the future. These changes may have an effect on the nursing profession, and will therefore require a willingness by the nurse to co-operate more closely with all members of the team. Not only is it necessary for the nurse to broaden her concept of a multidisciplinary team, but also to plan her nursing interventions to make maximum use of the contributions of members from other sectors of the team. This is imperative if the ultimate objective of assisting the community to achieve optimal health is to be realised.

3.6 SUMMARY

In view of the many pressing health issues facing the world today, the recognition and effective utilisation of all members of the multidisciplinary health care team by health care planners is long overdue.

The health system will have to be adaptive in nature, and must promote multidisciplinary and intersectoral action for health, based on the needs of all sectors of the community. There are, however, many barriers that will have to be overcome before such collaboration is successful.

A truly multidisciplinary, intersectoral health care team must be available to facilitate interaction to the benefit of the community, to collect information, mobilise resources and channel their activities in order to promote health for all. To achieve results that will benefit all sections of the community, the multidisciplinary health care team will have to:

- co-operate with all who can contribute to the health and well-being of the community
- promote community participation in health matters
- promote co-operation based on trust
- co-ordinate efforts of all the role-players in order to achieve synergistic results
- agree on definite goals, as well as on the means of achieving such goals
- share resources and information to the benefit of the community
- be acceptable to the community
- retain credibility
- fulfil an advocacy role on behalf of the community
- strive for the achievement of equality in health care
- remain flexible and open to new approaches to health care delivery.

Above all, the community health nurse, and all members of an effective multidisciplinary health care team, should always have as their ultimate objective, providing assistance to the community to attain the highest possible level of health and well-being.

Bibliography

African National Congress. 1992. ANC policy guidelines on health. *South African medical journal*. December, Vol. 82:392–3.

African National Congress. 1994. *A national health plan for South Africa.* Johannesburg: ANC.

Bernhard, L.A. and Walsh, M. 1990. *Leadership: the key to professionalization of nursing*. 2nd ed. St Louis: Baltimore.

Bury, J.A. and Svensson, P-G. (Eds) 1994. *Training and research in public health: policy perspectives for a "new public health"*. Karlstad: Centre for Public Health Research/WHO Collaborating Centre.

Chell, E. 1985. *Participation and organization: a social psychological approach.* London: Macmillan.

Clark, M.J.D. 1984. *Community health care for today and tomorrow.* Reston: Prentice-Hall.

Cooney, C. (Ed.) 1994. *Primary health care – the way to the future.* New York: Prentice Hall.

Department of National Health and Population Development. 1992. *Strategy* for primary health care in South Africa: report by Subcommittee on Primary Health Care. Pretoria: Government Printer.

Dreyer, M., Hattingh, S. and Lock, M. 1993. *Fundamental aspects in community health nursing*. Halfway House: Southern.

Glatthaar, E. 1990. Editorial comment. *CHASA journal of comprehensive health*. June, Vol. 1, No. 1:2.

Glatthaar, E. 1993. Editorial comment. *CHASA journal of comprehensive health*. Jan–Feb, Vol. 4, No. 1:2.

Goddard, J.M.M. 1983. The team concept in community health care. *Curationis*. December, Vol. 4:37–9.

Hammad, A.E.B. 1986. Intersectoral cooperation in primary health care. *World health*. March:3–5.

IJsselmuiden, C. 1993. The Transvaal School of Public Health: towards education for health. *CHASA journal of comprehensive health*. Vol. 4, No. 3:57–61.

Lightfoot, G.V. 1991. Working together as a team. *ITC communicator*. Jan–Feb:1.

Lock, M., Dreyer, J., Ferreira, M., Krynauw, J. and Dennill, K. 1992. *Community health nursing science: study guide 1 for CNU100-U (an introductory overview to community health and community health nursing science)*. Pretoria: University of South Africa.

Miller, J. 1995. Community partnerships make headway on three continents (Perspectives). *International journal of the WK Kellogg Foundation*. Vol. 6, No. 1:8–11.

Moji, N.C. 1990. Health care systems: organisation, options and opportunities. *CHASA journal of comprehensive health*. October, Vol. 1, No. 2:123–6.

Pick, W. 1992. Primary health care: some lessons for South Africa. *South African medical journal*. November, Vol. 82:300–1.

Poulton, B.C. and West, M.A. 1993. Effective multidisciplinary teamwork in primary health care. *Journal of advanced nursing*. Vol. 18:918–25.

Pritchard, P. 1981. *Manual of primary health care: its nature and organisation*. Oxford: Oxford University Press.

Roemer, M.I. 1988. Preparing public health leaders for the 1990s. *Public health reports*. Sept–Oct, Vol. 103, No. 5:443–52.

Stanhope, M.E. and Lancaster, J. 1992. *Community health nursing: process and practice for promoting health*. 3rd ed. St Louis: Mosby.

Van Rensburg, H.C.J., Fourie, A. and Pretorius, E. 1992. *Health care in South Africa: structure and dynamics*. Pretoria: Academica.

World Health Organisation. 1986. *Intersectoral action for health*. Geneva: WHO.

World Health Organisation. 1988. *Learning together to work together for health. Report of a WHO Study Group on multiprofessional education of health personnel: the team approach*. Technical report series No. 769. Geneva: WHO.

World Health Organisation. 1994. *Statements of Dr Hiroshi Nakajima, Director-General, to the Executive Board and the World Health Assembly*. Geneva: WHO.

Yach, D., Pick, W. and Padayachee, N. 1990. Critical issues for community health in South Africa in the 1990s. *CHASA journal of comprehensive health*. June, Vol. 1, No. 1:38–4.

4

Community participation in health care delivery

LAETITIA KING

CHAPTER OBJECTIVES

After reading this chapter, the student should be able to:

- discuss the concepts dealt with in this chapter
- compare, examine critically and analyse the different interpretations of the concept of community participation
- conceptualise the relationship between community development and community participation in health
- identify the obstacles that hinder community participation
- identify the ways in which the community can participate in the prevention of disease and the promotion of health
- list the advantages of community participation in health
- analyse the value of community participation in the prevention of disease and the promotion of health
- discuss how community participation in health can be facilitated
- explain the role of health professionals in promoting community participation and partnership
- outline strategies relevant to the development and management of community projects.

4.1 INTRODUCTION

Community participation in health care delivery is more than a basic requirement for the attainment of optimal health of the community. As a process of interaction between people to achieve specific goals, it not only gives them the right and opportunity to be involved in decisions that affect their future existence, but also ensures the successful development of the community as a whole. Okoro (1995:145) is of the opinion that the achievement of an appropriate health care delivery system will not be possible unless there is "involvement of all people including those at grassroots level". Cooney (1994:63), in turn, reminds us that "one of the cornerstones of democracy is the right of citizens to be involved in decisions that affect their lives", but appears to be somewhat sceptical about the success of such involvement, by adding that, although nobody would deny the legitimacy of the previous statement, the extent to which such involvement occurs, remains a controversial issue.

The urgency to develop community participation in health is reflected in the following statement put forth during the technical discussions at the forty-seventh World Health Assembly in Geneva in May 1994:

> ". . . the urgent need for community action for health arises from a combination of factors. On the one hand, the community has gradually come to realize its need and responsibility to assume a greater share of the initiative for its own health care. On the other hand, there has been a growing awareness among health care decision-makers that without community action, much-needed behavioural changes will not occur and opportunities to prevent major causes of mortality and morbidity will be missed (WHO 1994(a):8)".

In the process of involving the community in health care planning and related activities, it will often be found that there are marked differences in how the various members of the health team will perceive the implementation of the concept "community participation". Cooney (1994:62) suggests that the first step that the team should take is to "... explore their fundamental beliefs about the involvement of the public in health care and the values that are linked to those beliefs".

Support for the concept of community participation and democracy in health care delivery is professed by the majority of countries. There is, however, some scepticism with regard to the success of such support. The WHO Director-General, Dr Nakajima, refers to participation by the community in health related matters as "Community Action for Health",and maintains that it "implies a significant change in approach for both communities and government". He warns, however, that "a genuine partnership between the health system and the community has yet to evolve in many countries" (WHO 1994:2).

This concern is shared by Wilson *et al.* (1991:372), who maintain that community participation and democracy are ideals which can easily become empty slogans unless clarity regarding these concepts is established, for it has been found that the motivation to promote community participation, and the success with which it is implemented, could vary greatly.

As part of the African National Congress (ANC) policy guidelines on health, as adopted at a national conference on 28 to 31 May 1992, it was proposed that a comprehensive, equitable and integrated national health service (NHS) be created. The following statement, which, at that time, was included in the policy guidelines, highlights the importance with which the ANC views community participation in all aspects of health care provision (*SA Medical Journal* 1992:392): The NHS will actively promote community participation in the planning, provision, control and monitoring of services. Fundamental to this approach will be accountability to local communities and decentralisation of decision-making.

This commitment of the ANC to the PHC (Primary Health Care) approach in health care delivery, and to the promotion of community participation in such health care, has since become a reality. Chimere-Dan (1996:ix) states that "in South Africa community involvement in development programmes - including health programmes - is in line with international trends and also appears to be a legitimate response by those long excluded from decision-making in the political and economic spheres. The current initiative by the government to address South Africa's health problems regards community involvement as a principal ingredient".

In the White Paper for the transformation of the health system in South Africa (Government Gazette Notice 667 of 1997), it is stated that, in order to realise the mission and goals of the South African Health Sector, "it is envisaged that the National Health System (NHS) will incorporate all stakeholders, i.e. the government sector, NGOs (including religious and grassroots organisations), the private sector and, especially, the communities" (Department of Health 1997:13). It is also stated that it is essential that the active participation and involvement of all sectors of the South African society in health and health-related activities be obtained, and that the people of South Africa should realise that, without their active participation, little progress will be made in the process of improving their health status.

According to the Department of Health (1997:16), the South African health sector's goals and objectives include, *inter alia*, the following:

"***(f) To foster community participation across the health sector:***
- (i) involve communities in various aspects of the planning and provision of health services;
- (ii) establish mechanisms to improve public accountability and promote dialogue and feedback between the public and health providers; and
- (iii) encourage communities to take greater responsibility for their own health promotion and care."

4.2 EMPOWERMENT OF THE COMMUNITY

The concept of community participation in the delivery of health services must not only be acknowledged for its value with regard to the prevention of disease and the promotion of health. The role it plays in the empowerment of communities and the elimination of social inequalities is also of paramount importance. Commenting on community participation in health service institutions, Venter (1993:290) refers to the view held by Shisana and Versfeld that communities should be motivated to become involved, and that if such stimulation of the community is undertaken with a genuine desire to guide them towards becoming self-reliant, empowerment of the community will be achieved. Empowerment of a community to make decisions about its own affairs is defined by the Namibian Ministry of Health and Social Services (1992:19), as "the process where community members come together to share and discuss their problems and needs, prioritize them and find possible solutions which they then plan, implement and assess through continuous monitoring, dialogue and evaluation based on their objectives".

Gajanayake and Gajanayake (1993:6) describe empowerment as follows:

> "Empowerment is a concept that goes beyond participation. It implies enabling people to understand the reality of their environment, reflect on the factors shaping that environment, and take steps to effect changes to improve the situation. It is a process that encompasses people deciding where they are now, where they want to go, and developing and implementing plans to reach their goals, based on self-reliance and sharing of power. Most importantly, empowerment helps people to liberate themselves from mental and physical dependants. It is, in essence, the ability to stand independently, think progressively, plan and implement changes systematically, and accept the outcomes rationally."

4.3 CLARIFICATION OF CONCEPTS

Before the concept of community participation in health care delivery can be analysed, it is necessary to clarify various concepts relevant to the discussion.

4.3.1 Community

A community can be described in terms of its geographic boundaries or its social boundaries, or both (Dreyer *et al.* 1993:111). Agudelo, as cited by Woelk (1992:419), defines a community as a group of people who live in a particular area and who have shared values, cultural patterns and social problems, as well as a group awareness which facilitates the residents interacting more intensely with each other than they would with outsiders.

Alihonou *et al.* (1993:9) list three definitions cited by Rifkin *et al.*(1988), in which a community is defined firstly in terms of geographic boundaries, secondly simply as "a group of people sharing the same basic interests", and thirdly according to target groups, or "at-risk" groups in the community. Alihonou *et al.* also remind us that most definitions of the concept do not fully describe the complexities of a community, and warn that it is vital for health professionals who wish to promote community participation to remember that a "community is not simply composed of target populations or high risk groups who require positive action, but that there are other essential aspects which must be taken into account, if we want the community to become involved".

What is important, when defining a community, is to recognise the sharing of various aspects basic to the existence of the particular community, and the bond which develops between members of the community. Not only is the existence and acknowledgement of these factors crucial to the success or failure of community participation, but achieving equality in health care for the total community also depends on it. Empowerment of the community is therefore a vital factor in community participation.

4.3.2 Community participation and involvement

Community participation in health can be described as the active involvement of people who live together in some form of social organisation and cohesion, in the planning, operation and control of primary health care, by using local, national and other resources. Not only are the results of such participation of importance, but the process of participation in itself, also warrants attention.

According to the WHO (1994:15), participation can be classified as:

- marginal participation, where there is limited community input
- substantive participation, where the community is actively involved in priority determination
- structural participation, where active involvement of the community becomes the ideological basis for the project itself
- spontaneous participation, in which the community participates in local, self-sustaining initiatives which have little or no external support
- induced participation, which occurs where there are previously defined external initiatives which merely require community endorsement
- compulsory participation, which implies that communities are organised to participate in activities over which they have very little influence
- participation where community co-operation is actively sought by government before decisions are implemented
- community participation, such as power-sharing, where the community members have the right to participate in all decision-making, and may veto ideas which are contrary to the objectives of the community.

There are three basic characteristics to note in the concept of community participation, i.e. participation must be active, people have the right and responsibility to exercise power over decisions that affect their lives, and there must be mechanisms available to allow the implementation of the decisions made by the community. In line with these basic characteristics,

Rifkin *et al.* (1988:933) advocate that community participation is "a social process whereby specific groups with shared needs living in a defined geographic area actively pursue identification of their needs, take decisions and establish mechanisms to meet these needs".

Although the concept of community participation in health care is used in preference to community involvement in health care in this chapter, in the literature both concepts are used interchangeably to refer to the mechanism in which the community is acknowledged as a partner in the process of achieving optimal health for all.

Wall and Lischeron (1977:37) discuss involvement as an aspect of participation, and suggest that it "concerns the essentially interactive, constructive and problem-solving orientation of those involved". Chell (1985:1) says that from a social psychological point of view participation can also be defined in terms of involvement and influence, and refers to a study by Vroom who describes psychological participation as the "influence that an individual feels he has in decision-making". Wall and Lischeron (1977:36) also refer to the element of decision-making in participation, and suggest that participation is not a unitary concept, but that it consists of interrelated elements which manifest in decision-making processes. They maintain that influence, interaction and information-sharing are three elements central to the concept of participation. Vandervelde, in Kramer and Specht (1983:95), states that people should be involved in decisions which affect them, and places great emphasis on what she terms "participative decision making".

Brearly (1990:2) describes community participation, or patient participation, in terms of the following three components:

- self-help, meaning the patient is actively involved in care
- demedicalisation, meaning professional care is substituted by lay care
- democratisation, meaning consumers are involved in social policy decisions regarding health care.

Self-help often takes place by means of group activities. Such self-help groups can be defined as follows:

> "Self-help groups are voluntary, small group structures for mutual aid and the accomplishment of a special purpose. They are usually founded by peers who have come together for mutual assistance in satisfying a common need, overcoming a common handicap or life-disrupting problem and bringing about desired social and/or personal change." (Brearly 1990:19)

Self-help groups have a strong tradition in South Africa, and according to Van Rensburg *et al.* (1992:345), can be divided into the following four categories:

- self-help groups which are an extension of the activities of the health professions

- self-help groups whose aim is to promote the interests of clients/patients
- self-help groups which summarily reject professional health workers or any offer of help
- self-help groups with no interest in professional health workers or their services.

The value of self-help efforts with regard to health care issues cannot be disputed. However, it is necessary to not only view community participation in health from the perspective of what the individual in the community can do towards improving her or his own health in this regard, but to also consider how the individual can co-operate with the professional health team in other ways towards improving the health of the wider community.

Of particular significance in the various definitions of community participation is the constant referral to the need to allow the community to be part of the decision-making process. The overall message is that, only once the community has the right and opportunity to participate in the actual decision-making processes which affect health care, will community participation be truly democratic. This approach is supported by the view of Shisana and Versfeld (1993:6), who describe effective community participation in terms of successful power-sharing. They also express the opinion that community partnership involves a negotiated relationship in which both service and community organisations accept the responsibility to perform tasks that have been agreed upon to enable the community to achieve its objectives. With regard to the suggested power component, some authors refer to power-sharing and power-equalisation in decision-making. Vandervelde (in Kramer and Specht 1983:99) maintains, however, that although power equalisation refers to the reduction of power exerted by some people, it would not be wise always to equate participation with power equalisation. The emphasis should indeed be on sharing. Organisational decision-making, as referred to in Kramer and Specht (1983:96), should be seen on a continuum, from a totally authoritarian approach to a fully delegated one. The cost of endless discussions that lead nowhere must be kept in mind, and they should be avoided. Decision-making should be a joint effort with strong goal orientation and standards, as well as specific constraints. According to Vandervelde (in Kramer and Specht 1983:96), "certain areas of responsibility and accountability can and must be retained for the manager without compromising the participative process".

The various interpretations of community involvement and participation that have been discussed can be summarised as follows:

- people's involvement in decision-making processes

- their involvement in implementing programmes and decisions by contributing various resources or co-operation in specific organisations or activities
- their sharing in the benefits of development programmes
- their involvement in efforts to evaluate such programmes.

What is clear from all the definitions is that community participation, to be effective, must be a collaborative effort, must acknowledge the importance of power-sharing, allow community involvement in decision-making processes and assist the community in the achievement of equality in health.

4.3.3 Community development

No discussion on community participation can be complete without discussion of the concept of community development. Community participation, or involvement, is a vital part of community development, while it can also be said that community development is a natural result of community participation. It is also true that any attempt at establishing community development must include the development of the people, which means that the community, by participating in such efforts, plays an active part in its own development. The community should therefore also understand that not participating has a negative effect on its own development. Democratisation of the management of development programmes, according to Shisana and Versfeld (1993:5), is ensured through involvement of the community.

Mayfield (1985:xiii), in discussing the challenge of rural development programmes, refers to a process of rural reconstruction, and maintains that it in fact requires the "liberation of the human spirit". He continues by stating that, whereas rural development projects can change many things in a community, unless the people themselves change, self-sustaining development will be very difficult. Bjaras, Haglund and Rifkin (1991:204) refer to the change that occurs due to community participation in health projects, and state: "Community intervention is a strategy based on the concept that the process inherent in community participation actually changes community norms and values regarding the health problem being addressed".

Dr James Yen (Mayfield 1985:viii) worked among the illiterate poor of China during the first half of this century. The lessons that can be learned from his experiences and wisdom are immense, and can even today be applied with great benefit to any attempt at community development. The basic message of this remarkable man is that "if you want to help the poor, first you must go to them and learn from them". He also maintained that the poor have many potential powers waiting for release, not relief. Although it is today more acceptable to talk of empowerment, the need to help the community to achieve such release is as relevant today as it has ever been. In addition to community empowerment, the shift should be away from giving advice to the community, to promoting community decision-making.

Mayfield (1985:16) also suggests that community development should be approached in a systematic way, since economic problems are usually closely related to social and political systems, educational programmes cannot be divorced from health programmes and cultural values will greatly influence all organisational efforts.

The following broad principles are suggested by Bopape (1980:36) as basic to the concept of community development:

- mutual involvement of government and the people is necessary to initiate community development
- community co-operation must be stimulated and enhanced, not forced
- only projects relevant to the needs of the community should be developed, because the community will be more willing to identify with such projects
- human dignity must be respected by involving the people in decisions that affect them
- to ensure that projects can be sustained, attention must be given to the long-term changes that take place in the attitudes of people
- existing grassroots organisations should be utilised where possible
- development must be accompanied by education of the people
- central assistance may be required where needs cannot be met by small-scale action
- both economic and social development should be attended to in community development initiatives
- community development requires intersectoral action, since it produces multidimensional effects.

Successful community development will only be achieved if there is commitment from all concerned, and the approach is based on the needs and priorities of the community. All activities should be implemented with their full participation and involvement. The community must be supported in its efforts to achieve its objectives, which should allow maximum community responsibility and accountability for its development programmes in a spirit of self-reliance and self-determination. To ensure that community development contributes towards the achievement of optimal health for all, it is necessary to actively promote community participation in health matters.

(a) Strategies relevant to the development and management of community projects

A community development project can be defined as an initiative aimed at improving the quality of life of disadvantaged people. It should assist with the development of the community, and should consider carefully how it can meet the actual needs of the people in a sustainable way.

Gajanayake and Gajanayake (1993:7) developed a comprehensive and systematic model to follow in the planning, implementation and evaluation of community development projects. The model, which includes maximum community participation, incorporates seven major steps which ultimately assist in generating and implementing solutions to address identified community needs, while at the same time contributing towards community empowerment. The seven steps are:

- Understanding the community (community assessment)
- Needs assessment and prioritisation
- Determination of goals and objectives
- Assessment of available resources and anticipated constraints
- Planning project activities
- Implementation of the project
- Evaluation of project outcomes.

The schematic outline presented in Figure 4.1 summarises the community project development model suggested by Gajanayake and Gajanayake.

Community development projects require careful planning and systematic approaches to ensure the effective implementation and desired outcomes of the projects. As part of the planning process, a clear project proposal should be written as the first step in ensuring the ultimate success of the project, and it is important that community development agents will develop the skills required in order to write effective project proposals.

A project proposal is a concise document that provides a clear idea of what the particular project is all about, and should at least indicate the following:

- what specific strategies are being considered for the implementation of the project
- who will benefit from the project
- how the project will operate
- what the requirements are for the effective implementation of the project.

Swanepoel and De Beer (1996(b)), discuss the importance of writing effective project proposals and indicate that a project proposal not only forms the basis for fundraising, but also provides guidelines according to which the progress of the project can be monitored, and the outcomes thereof can be evaluated.

FIGURE 4.1 : Community project development model

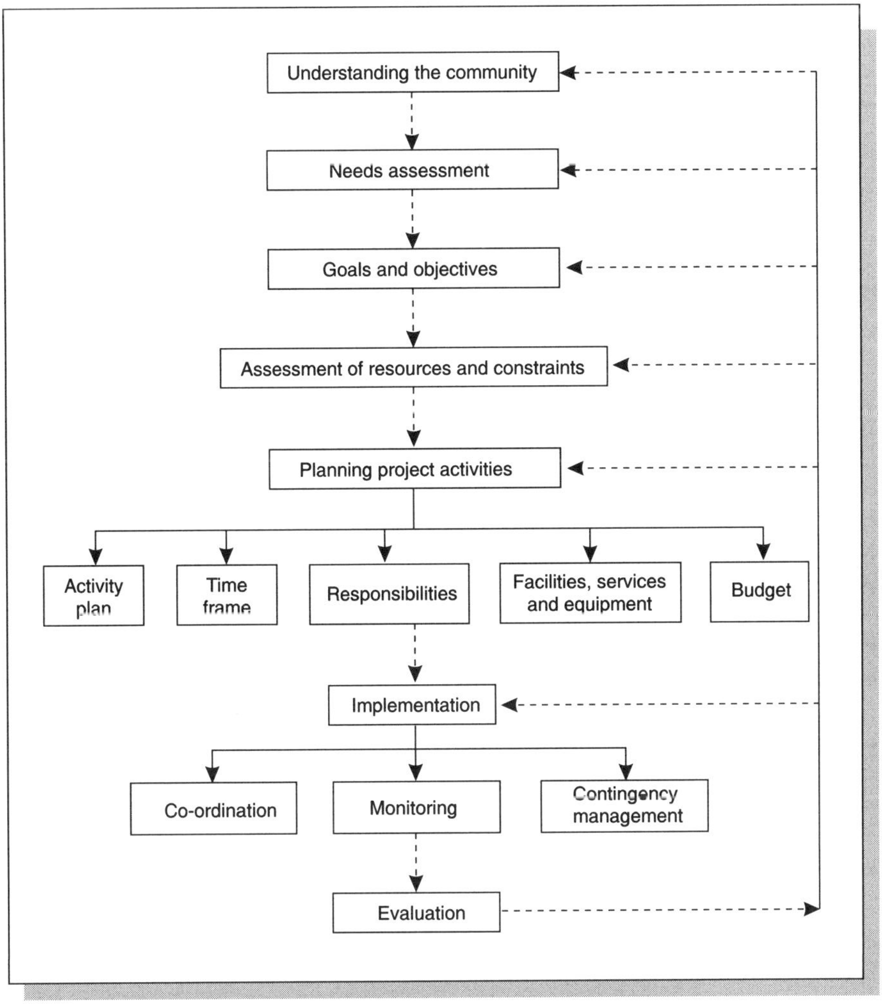

Source: Gajanayake and Gajanayake (1993.7)

A good project should have clear objectives and a well-planned timetable. Although the aims and objectives of projects could be as varied as the needs that the various projects may have to address, it can be assumed that a good community project should at least be able to:

- satisfy identified needs
- contribute to quality of life
- develop a sense of ownership among the community members

- promote community involvement in the project and related activities
- stimulate community contribution on all levels
- be done *with* the community and not *for* the community
- involve excellent planning and control
- ensure sustainability of the project.

4.4 DIFFERENT INTERPRETATIONS OF THE CONCEPT OF COMMUNITY PARTICIPATION IN HEALTH

Although community participation is generally accepted as a vital component of effective public health care, the effectiveness and value of the concept have not always been viewed in the same way by all concerned. Vuori (1984:331) maintains that not only are there different interpretations of the concept, but that there is in fact "no agreement on who participates in what; and, in spite of public lip service, the true attitudes may be hostile". However, as is evident from the previous discussion reflecting the commitment of the Department of Health and others towards the concept of community participation, there can be no doubt that community participation is a vital component of any attempt at achieving optimal health for all.

According to Rifkin and Cassels (1990:39), community participation can be interpreted in one of the following ways:

- *compliance*: people are motivated to accept interventions, or to act according to the advice of professionals
- *contribution*: the community supplements the contributions of professionals
- *collaboration*: the community participates in planning and introducing initiatives
- *control*: the community oversees the activities and manages the resources.

The views most often expressed about the approach towards community participation can be broadly categorised as being community participation with either hidden or open agendas.

There are those who believe that the state promotes community participation merely to co-opt people to provide a service which it is unable or unwilling to provide itself. In such a view the promotion of community partnership is seen as oppressive and with various hidden agendas. Wilson *et al.* (1991:372) refer to the traditional description of community participation in primary health care as it relates to the extent to which the community members give freely of their time, their labour and their money towards "their" health service. The authors describe poor rural people involved in building and running their own health centres, and warn that not only is it the responsibility of governments to build health centres, but that "the democratic rights of health workers who have their own needs and interests must not be confused with the democratic rights of the community".

A more acceptable approach to community participation is one in which the community, as part of the multidisciplinary health care team, is involved in the planning, provision and control of health services. The community members should participate in identifying health needs and priorities, and should agree on the nature of their personal contribution towards solving their identified problems. The community must be able to make rational decisions regarding health approaches to its own circumstances. This approach to participation, a community-supportive approach, will supplement and complement government health services to the benefit of the community without reducing the value of existing services.

4.5 COMMUNITY REPRESENTATION BY NON-GOVERNMENTAL ORGANISATIONS

In addition to official governmental activities in health and related matters, there are many non-governmental organisations (NGOs) that represent communities in matters of importance to their health and well-being, and which warrant active community participation. It is also suggested that there are many other development stakeholders ranging, *inter alia*, from civic to church and women's organisations, and from youth groups to taxi-owners and shebeen associations. Although there is general recognition of the need for strong community organisations in a democratic South African community, the following statement suggests that such organisations may need to undergo certain changes in the future (Bernstein and McCarthy 1994:79):

> "The enormous transition away from an apartheid society and towards a democratic one involves a fundamental reassessment of all the institutions of our society. Some are strong and must be built upon for the future; some must change and play a new role; and some must die as their particular function is no longer needed or relevant in a democratic system."

It is suggested that the relationship of NGOs with government and programmes such as the RDP could have the following consequences:

- NGOs can influence policy development through an assessment of community needs and feeding these needs to government
- NGOs can help bridge the communication gap between communities and government
- NGOs can advise government by assisting in the monitoring of programmes such as the RDP

- NGOs can ensure quick delivery of development activities as they are not hamstrung by bureaucracy
- NGOs can bring their experience and expertise to the implementation of government initiated programmes.

It is generally accepted that NGOs can assist communities in various ways. These organisations can, for instance, assist communities in the development of the required capacity to control their own development and, in addition, can help them to define their own needs and priorities. Community participation in government-initiated programmes can be facilitated through the efforts of NGOs, and in that way the attention of the government can be drawn to the problems of the community.

4.6 OBSTACLES TO COMMUNITY PARTICIPATION

Although most health care workers in South Africa would attest to the importance of community participation, acceptance of the concept is not shared by all health team members with the same enthusiasm. Shisana and Versfeld (1993:5) write, "While the concept of community participation is now several years old for those working in non-governmental progressive health organisations, it is relatively new to many mainstream health service organisations." It is also necessary to take note of the many negative attitudes expressed by an increasing number of individuals, who bear witness to many failed attempts at promoting community participation and yet succumb to increasing pressure to promote it.

In addition to the fact that most communities are not entirely homogeneous, and thus would not necessarily always be willing or able to participate co-operatively in efforts to improve their health and well-being, there are various other obstacles to effective community participation that should be avoided or, should they occur, addressed. Shisana and Versfeld (1993:6) note the following factors that could adversely affect community participation: "the history of the health service with the community, the belief system and culture, and experience with other similar institutions which have generated mistrust and negative pressure groups". Inadequate organisational support to involve the community in health care, as well as financial or geographic maldistribution of health care services, will also have a negative effect on community participation. Robb *et al.* (1991:372) maintain that "it makes no sense to talk of either community participation or democracy in health when health care is beyond the financial or geographical reach of the majority of the people". They also make the point that community participation will be of no value as long as "control lies in the hands of rich and privileged professionals and the ownership of multinational corporations". Farley (1993:244) recognised this obstacle: "bureaucracies and health professionals are often not eager to relinquish power and control, or to engage in activities that will infringe on their status and privileges." Certain health service providers are reluctant to promote community self-reliance as they see it as a threat to their power base. Such misuse of power is bound to lead to conflict between the services and the community.

Community participation will not be successful unless the professional members of the multidisciplinary health team accept the community as active members of the team, and not as a threat to their positions. This also holds true for political decision-makers who, rather than suppress community involvement out of fear of loss of power, should utilise the available expertise to improve the health and well-being of the community. Vuori (1984:12) is of the opinion that "at the heart of this issue is the right balance between vesting enough power in the governors to govern, while still enabling the governed to exercise final control and engage in effective involvement in the process of governing". On the other hand, there is a belief that at times community participation is used as a ploy by politicians to achieve political gain. A report of the Kaiser Family Foundation, as cited by Shisana and Versfeld (1993:6), warns that "there is a risk that the whole concept of community participation is being perverted in South Africa at present to suit the short-term ends of political actors". Furthermore, the statement by Shisana and Versfeld (1993:7) that the South African health services are still associated by many community members with the apartheid government, and that this leads to tension and lack of trust between the health services and the community, is a further indication of how community attitudes towards official health services can adversely affect community participation. The political situation in a community can have a marked effect on community participation.

Although some authors draw attention to the fact that a common history of struggle in a community could mobilise its members towards community participation, Woelk (1992:422) reminds us of the potential difficulties to sustain such participation: "The struggle is a continuing one, for it involves constant pressure to ensure a more equitable distribution of resources, in the face of bureaucratisation and circulating elites, where there are changes in the leaders but not necessarily in the structure of the leadership." The current political situation in South Africa gives much reason to question the sustainability of community participation. There are situations where only passive participation in projects occurs, because they are perceived to be government-linked. This is usually ascribed to situations where the political environment is not conducive to community involvement. It is, however, also necessary to keep in mind that the culture of violence, which appears to be the order of the day, makes community participative efforts not only difficult, but in certain areas virtually impossible.

Sekgobela (1986:30) maintains that differing cultural practices and communication problems between the community and the health care providers often present obstacles to community participation. She writes that the community might not know what it wants, or could be reluctant to become involved due to previously unfulfilled expectations. All these obstacles point to a lack of information being made available to the community, and highlight the need for improved health education as a basic requirement for effective community participation. It is important to note the warning by Shisana and Versfeld (1993:8) that "unless community involvement has a strong educational component, the involvement will not be sustained".

Obstacles to community participation are not only associated with the health professionals or the health care system. Many reasons for inadequate or ineffective participation can be attributed to the community. At times communities might lack the necessary leadership to promote participation, but general apathy, and a hesitancy by individuals in the community to volunteer their time, money or energy, might also have a negative influence on participation. Incorrect assumptions about community participation must be eliminated, by both health professionals, who need to accept the community as part of the team, and the individual community members who might not be aware of all the implications associated with community participation in health. The community and the health professionals need to recognise the costs associated with participation in terms of time, effort and money.

4.7 ADVANTAGES OF COMMUNITY PARTICIPATION

Although attention must be given to eliminating the obstacles to community participation, recognition should also be given to the many benefits that can be attributed to involving the community on a partnership basis in aspects that influence their health and well-being.

The effectiveness of community participation in the prevention of disease and the promotion of health varies from one community to another. According to Sekgobela (1986:30), support for community participation in health activities is, however, not unanimous. She maintains that some people avoid involving the community on the basis of their alleged ignorance, while others are uncertain as to how or when the community should be involved. Acknowledging various obstacles, Sekgobela nevertheless lists the following advantages of community participation:

- Through community participation the health team can obtain first-hand information about local conditions and needs.

- Community members will be more committed to community projects if they are involved in the planning, preparation and maintenance of projects they consider important.
- Community participation gives the community an opportunity to exercise its democratic right to be involved in its own development.
- Through participation the community will become more self-reliant, self-sufficient, self-confident and independent.
- Through joint discussions between the health planners and the people, power differences and potential corruption are reduced.
- Planning is more likely to be done according to local circumstances and available resources if the community is involved.
- Community participation supplements community services.

The advantages of community involvement in health, as outlined by the WHO (1991), can be summarised as follows:

- Community involvement is a basic right of all people.
- Involvement in the decisions and actions affecting people's health builds up self-esteem and encourages a sense of responsibility.
- Through community involvement limited resources can be applied more appropriately to satisfy needs as identified by the local community, and can complement and supplement formal health services.
- Community involvement in health can help to create political awareness, encouraging people to get involved in other areas of development of the community.

Vuori (1984:338) draws attention to the psychological and material benefits that participation holds for the individual. Psychological benefits relate to the satisfaction derived from fulfilling a civic duty, while material benefits are obtained as a result of the decisions which one has influenced through participation. Involvement in decision-making gives community members a sense of control over their lives, and thereby promotes social justice. Through participation, co-operation between the members of the community is developed, allowing them, through their acceptance of responsibility and accountability for activities, to develop self-reliance. This enables the community to make a meaningful contribution towards the achievement of equality in health. Ferrinho (1993) maintains that participation can be expressed as the principle of human solidarity, which he says "is not only a moral responsibility manifested through intentions but also a social responsibility which imposes, as a duty, the participation in the making and implementation of decisions about public affairs".

A further advantage of participation relates to the personal benefit or satisfaction that the individual derives from community togetherness. As social beings, humans need to relate closely to the members of the community to which they belong. Community participation, if practised effectively, not only achieves the primary objectives of such involvement, but also satisfies people's need for belonging and togetherness.

The advantages of community participation in health that have been listed, are echoed in the following three interpretations of the concept of community participation given by Shisana and Versfeld (1993:6):

- Community participation allows the community an opportunity to contribute towards predetermined programmes.
- Through community participation the community obtains representation in organisational structures, leading to power-sharing among participants.
- Community participation results in empowerment of the community to make decisions about its own affairs.

4.8 FACILITATING COMMUNITY PARTICIPATION

To suggest an ideal approach for the achievement of effective community participation is unrealistic. The cultural background, availability of human and other resources in the health system, educational facilities available to the health team and the general community, as well as the level of literacy of the community, will all influence the approach. If community participation is to contribute towards achieving community empowerment and general community development, it must be approached holistically, recognising the complexity of the community, and at the same time respecting its culture and uniqueness. Attention should not only be given to the material development of the community, but also to the social and spiritual dimensions of belonging to a "community". Vuori (1984:333) states that there cannot be one universal approach to community participation, and warns that community participation approaches must be tailored to the needs and cultural values of the particular country.

Shisana and Versfeld (1993:6) acknowledge that there is a strong and growing movement towards community participation, particularly among progressive non-governmental and civic organisations and health service providers in South Africa, but add that, although it is generally accepted that community participation is desirable, it is not clear how the communities should be involved. If it is accepted that participation means active involvement of the community in particular activities with shared control over their outcomes, the challenge that faces health workers is to motivate the community to embark on such activities, and then to network with the broader constituency.

In addition to active involvement of the community members, community participation will only be effective if there is political commitment and accountability, as well as adequate economic resources to sustain the process. Partnership between the public and private sector must be developed. Recognition and acceptance of civic organisations, and their contribution towards facilitating community participation, are necessary. Furthermore, it is important that both governmental and non-governmental organisations recognise each other's legitimate role and co-operate towards developing an effective partnership.

Many factors need to be considered before deciding on the most appropriate approach to establishing community participation in health.

4.8.1 Prerequisites for effective community participation

Anderson (1990:143) states that the following questions should be answered before co-operative involvement of people and their organisations in community development programmes can be secured.

- What are the specific tasks that are to be achieved?
- What is the nature of the required involvement?
- What contribution is required from the individuals and organisations involved?
- What is in it for them, for you, and for the community?

The following vital prerequisites for effective community participation in health can be suggested:

- a clear, stable and supportive national policy and political framework, characterised by political accountability and control, as well as effective management approaches
- community cohesion and commitment
- co-ordinated local intersectoral health programmes
- availability of a basic infrastructure (facilities and staff), as well as the required logistical support
- acceptance by all concerned of the multidimensional nature of the extended health team, which acknowledges the community as an active member of the team
- mutual support between the government and the community, reinforced by mutual information feedback
- clarity about the health and related needs of the community
- effective integration of health into overall community development
- recognition of socio-economic contradictions
- involvement of the community in the control of financial, human and other resources necessary for the provision of health services.

In addition to these prerequisites, careful planning, and the co-ordinated involvement of skilled people in project implementation, will be necessary to facilitate and sustain effective community participation. Shisana and Versfeld (1993:8) put it in a nutshell by stating that "community participation does not just occur, it must be developed through deliberate and skilful processes".

The processes to facilitate community participation should at least include the issues discussed below.

4.8.2 Community-based research and data collection

Adequate information about the community must be collected before community participation strategies can be promoted. Community-based research, including the collection of data regarding the nature of the community, its needs and priorities, as well as information about available community resources and facilities, must be undertaken before community participation can be facilitated. Bopape (1980:31) states that community involvement is a vital requirement for community development, and that it will only be effective if prior research is conducted regarding community spirit, leadership, cultural assets and social structure, as well as about internal and external systems. Tumwine (1989:158) feels that communities must be consulted when information is collected about their conditions, and warns health workers not to be paternalistic, but to acknowledge the wealth of knowledge that most community members have about their culture, the environment they live in, their needs, likes and dislikes, and the causes of ill health. The team that will be involved in the community health and development programmes must be carefully selected and adequately prepared. Specific health interventions, as well as the opportunities for community participation in such interventions, must be identified according to the specific needs and priorities of the community.

4.8.3 Initial contact and trust-building

Contact must be made with the community from the start, and a process of building trust must be initiated and continued. It is important to spend sufficient time during the initial contact stages building a strong foundation based on trust. Tumwine (1989:159) reminds us that "working in partnership with communities in order to help them improve their health is time-consuming, and needs a lot of patience and tact". This process of trust building must be continued and reinforced during regular meetings and workshops with the community.

4.8.4 Identification of community representatives

Community decision-making bodies, such as the civic and health committees within the community, must be identified and consulted. Vuori (1984:336) states that nomination of representatives by special interest groups could result in biased representation, while election or appointment by the authorities is just as unacceptable. Community representatives and leaders must, however, be identified in one way or another, ensuring that they are not self-appointed spokespersons, but are selected and accepted by the community. Democratically elected community groups such as the civic organisations, or local representative organisations such as church or youth groups from within the community, could also represent the community.

Community participation must be viewed in the context of representation and accountability. Although representation might appear to be a straightforward and obvious requirement for community participation, it is, in fact, quite a complex issue. It is not possible for an entire community to be actively involved in planning or decision-making activities. A representative body of the community must therefore be formed. The characteristics to be represented must be clearly specified, as must the interests that will be looked after. There should not only be descriptive representation, but also substantive representation, meaning that representatives act in the interests of those whom they represent (Kramer and Specht 1983:132). For substantive representation to be effective, accountability is a vital necessity. Attention must be given to the development of the leadership abilities of the representatives.

The representative, or working group, must be able to develop the programmes in which they become involved, in such a way that they will be compatible with the community philosophy, and yet achieve the objectives of the programme. This requires effort and commitment from all involved, for community action, according to Ferrinho (1993:35), "is in large measure conditioned by the levels of mental and physical energy which the people involved are able to invest in it".

4.8.5 Leadership development

A leadership development training programme that will assist local leaders to develop autonomy must be made available in the community. Mayfield (1985:131), in discussing the importance of leadership development in achieving effective community participation, states that local leadership and community participation require an interactive, self-sustaining process which he describes as the windmill effect. He maintains that the leadership aspect provides the energy that initiates and develops community participation activities and, in effect, is similar to the wind that is required to turn the blades of a windmill.

FIGURE 4.2 : The windmill effect

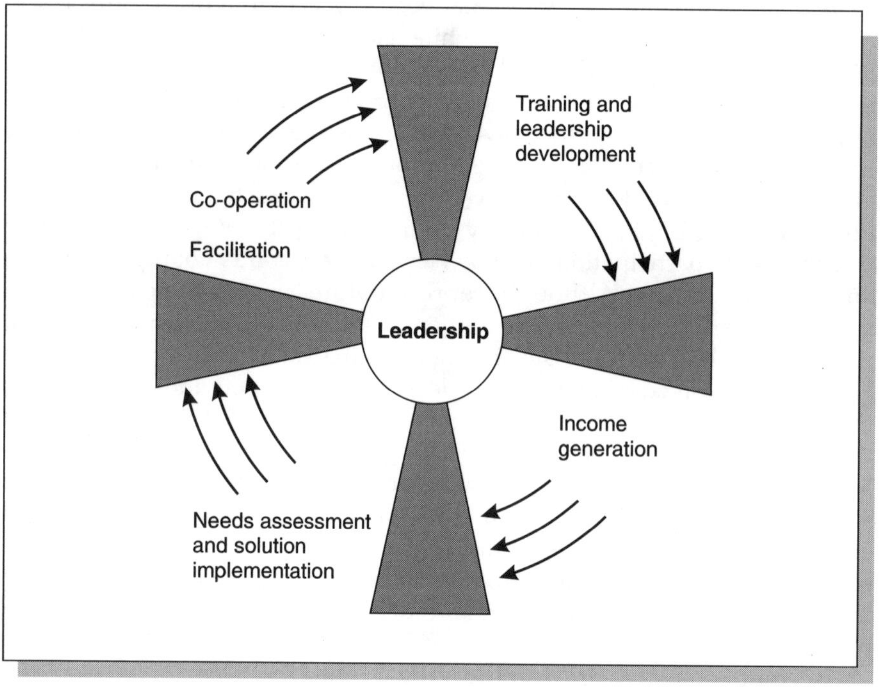

Source: Mayfield (1985:131)

The importance of leadership as a requirement for effective teamwork was addressed in some detail in the previous chapter.

4.8.6 Getting the message across: setting up workshops and public meetings

Shisana and Versfeld (1993:8) refer to the importance of "awareness-building" among the members of the community, in order to secure effective community participation. The community must be made aware of the importance of health and of health-related problems in the community. Agreement must be reached with the community on acceptable strategies for tackling the problems. This process of consultation and negotiation must commence in the initial stages of any attempt at facilitating community participation. Community projects, in which the community participates fully, will only be successful if adequate consultation with the community has taken place from the outset.

Acknowledging that community projects should satisfy felt needs of the community, Farley (1993:247) adds another dimension to this issue by stating that professionals can at times "serve to generate, channel and support community thought, concern, and action", because citizens might not always appreciate the intensity of their own needs, or may feel incapable of addressing such needs effectively.

4.8.7 Identification of the strengths of the community

The community must be guided to discover its own strengths and weaknesses, and to develop confidence in its own abilities. This view is supported by Farley (1993:247), who adds that the community's sense of confidence in directing its own efforts is essential to maintaining community participation. If effective community participation in health is to be sustained, due recognition must be given to the many strengths and areas of expertise present in the community. Health professionals must also accept that at times it might be necessary to ask the community for help. In this regard Wilson *et al.* (1991:373) refer to the community of Alexandra, which successfully assisted the local health centre personnel to mount a short and intensive immunisation campaign in the township during the 1986 polio epidemic that occurred there.

4.8.8 Identification of, and co-operation with, other projects in the community

If the provision of comprehensive health care is to become a reality, support must be given to all projects that actively promote the improvement of the health and well-being of the community. Such an approach is referred to by Wilson *et al.* (1991:373) as "extension work", such as the Alexandra Health Centre supporting other community projects and initiatives that are in some way involved with health and development in the local community. Shoo (1991:58) stresses the importance of what he calls "outreach activities", such as immunisation campaigns, or occasions when the health team assists a rural community with pressing local tasks such as weeding and harvesting.

4.8.9 Ongoing education to promote community participation

It is crucial to effective community participation that not only the health workers, but the community as well, be trained and retrained, so that they become competent in the participatory processes, and continue to feel confident as members of the team.

Shisana and Versfeld (1993:7) are of the opinion that "the ideals of self-reliance and empowerment are foreign both to members of the community, who have become used to being passive recipients of services, and health workers who expect to serve". In a similar vein Wilson *et al.* (1991:372) state that health workers must also learn to participate with the community, and emphasise how the health workers can participate in what the community is doing, and not only the other way round. According to Farley (1993:244), community participation refers to the establishment of true partnerships between health professionals and community members in order to allow the sharing of power and decision-making.

This is quite a daunting task, and to achieve success, professional health care workers need to learn how to appreciate power-sharing and decision-making with individuals in the community. Farley (1993:247) highlights the need for training all role-players in the participatory process, by stating that not only should investment in the development of human resources precede any project development, but that continuous formal and informal leadership training should be acknowledged as the key to sustaining community participation and to building successful coalitions. To ensure therefore that the community as a whole benefits from this knowledge base, the health team needs to tap into the vast knowledge and experience of the individuals in the community by involving them, and co-operating with them as full partners in the multidisciplinary health team.

In recognition of the value of increased consumer knowledge, training programmes aimed specifically at the community should, *inter alia,* give attention to the following aspects:

- Health promotion sessions regarding all aspects that influence the health and well-being of the community.
- Sessions aimed at creating a community awareness of the responsibilities of the community for improving and maintaining their own health and well-being.
- Sessions aimed at enlightening the community regarding the composition and activities of the extended multidisciplinary intersectoral health team, and how they, the community members, can become active partners in the team.
- Specific skills training sessions aimed at improving the abilities of the community to participate as members of the extended multidimensional health team in activities aimed at the empowerment of the community, social upliftment and health improvement. Relevant sessions in this regard should attend to leadership development, communication skills, interpersonal skills, transcultural understanding, skills in initiating and maintaining community projects, and so forth.

Health care training programmes should be largely community-based, and geared to develop the capabilities of all role-players to initiate and stimulate community participation in health. According to the WHO (1993:25), the training of all health workers should include field exposure to ensure that innovative approaches, applicable to the particular community, are included in the training programmes.

However, before the concept of community participation can be effectively dealt with in the training programmes, it is necessary to ensure that the concepts of teamwork and multidisciplinary, intersectoral co operation are clearly understood and accepted by all team members.

To ensure the successful implementation of a new health system in South Africa, based on the primary health care approach, health professionals will have to recognise that success depends not only on their involvement, but on the participation of all sectors of the community in health-related activities.

4.9 THE TRAINING OF HEALTH PROFESSIONALS TO PROMOTE COMMUNITY PARTICIPATION

Optimal health for all will not be possible without a concerted multidisciplinary, intersectoral team effort, which includes involvement of the community. Health professionals must promote such involvement by acknowledging the community as members of the team, and by motivating and assisting the community to accept the challenge of participation. Health care workers must accept the right of the community to participate actively in health care, and the community in turn must accept the responsibility that accompanies this right.

In order to assist the community in the process of becoming involved in health related matters, it is vital that health personnel are transformed in terms of their attitudes, behaviour, skills and knowledge. This requires not only a transformation of the health system, but it is necessary that the educational system should similarly be transformed.

The daunting task of transforming the South African educational system is being attended to by the National Commission for Higher Education (NCHE). A report on a proposed Framework for Transformation was published in October 1996, in which reference is made to a transformed higher education system which includes, *inter alia,* the concept of a National Qualifications Framework (NQF). These developments will have far-reaching effects on both general education and health worker training in South Africa. According to the commission, the proposed new educational system

> "... is underpinned by the key principles of equity, democratisation, development, quality, academic freedom/institutional autonomy, effectiveness and efficiency. Its three central features are increased participation by a diverse range of constituencies, increased co-operation and more partnerships between

higher education and other social actors and institutions, and greater responsiveness to social and economic needs" (NCHE 1996:i).

Although acknowledging the positive contribution of existing health personnel education and training approaches to public health care in South Africa, the 1996 NCHE report discusses the negative effects of the current system, and refers, *inter alia*, to earlier commissions, namely those of Loram (1928) and Gluckman (1942-44), in which factors such as "... the inappropriateness of health personnel training and its mismatch with national needs" are emphasised. Based on the government's support for a primary health care approach to health care delivery, the NCHE proposes that health worker education should be such that the members of the team will be capable of giving effect to the PHC approach in the NHS (NCHE 1996:342-343).

The need to adjust current approaches to health worker education in such a way that it satisfies the needs of the developing district-based health system of South Africa, is strongly supported by the NCHE. A district health system can be described as a system that

> "... refers to the devolved organisation of health services within a geographically defined area, mirroring local authority boundaries and which integrates community, primary, secondary and tertiary health care. It is linked to wider developmental and intersectoral initiatives around water, sanitation, etc. It is thus a strategy of organising health services which is development-directed, community-oriented and needs-based" (NCHE 1996:343).

A review of the approach to training and education is required in order to ensure that health care students and health personnel educators are equipped with the knowledge, competence and attitude to respond comprehensively and caringly to the health needs of the population.

Various local and international authors refer to the importance of teamwork and intersectoral co-operation in the training programmes of all health workers. In this regard the WK Kellogg Foundation maintains that serious attention needs to be given to curriculum changes of all health personnel regarding the multidisciplinary approach, in order to ensure that they are adequately prepared for community partnership initiatives. The need for a change to more community-based multidisciplinary training is highlighted, for, it is pointed out, "... seldom in traditional curricula do medical, nursing, and other health professions students have any common educational experience during their training" (Richards 1993:223).

IJsselmuiden (1993:68) supports the importance and value of multidisciplinary training, as can be deduced from the following comments with regard to professional development of members of the health team:

> "Typically, health-related education and research takes place within the narrow realm of single professions. Current education in public health is such that

> doctors set standards for doctors and doctors are trained by doctors. This applies equally to nurses, dentists, and environmental health officers. This type of training is inappropriate to deal with public health as a whole, as public health problems invariably require multidisciplinary and multisectoral solutions."

The multidisciplinary approach to the training of health workers is referred to by the NCHE as transdisciplinary work, and is defined as "... the intellectual endeavour to find solutions to problems which do not belong to a specific disciplinary field of academic inquiry, and which need a conceptual framework and methodological procedures that transcend the boundaries of traditional discipline" (NCHE1996:274).

Attending to the health manpower needs of a country, however, is not an easy task. Shoo (1991:61), in discussing the training of health workers in Tanzania, warns that merely increasing the number of health workers in a community will not necessarily improve the health of the community. He adds that "most government plans [in Tanzania] have concentrated on the numbers of health workers to be trained, whereas the aim should be to train health workers in such a way that they can mobilize their communities to improve their own health".

Health care workers need to develop a variety of skills to facilitate community participation, as well as the ability to teach these skills to people at grassroots level, to whom the concept of community participation may be quite foreign. Chell (1985:257) is of the opinion that people can be taught the skills necessary to cope with participative situations, and refers specifically to aspects such as being able to reduce stress and anxiety, to know when to make requests and when to give commands and how to disclose information. She adds, however, that to acquire such skills a great deal of thought and practice are necessary, since the skills incorporate both cognitive and affective elements. Shisana and Versfeld (1993:7) maintain: "A socio-anthropological understanding of communities, communication skills to facilitate dialogue with communities and an understanding of group dynamics are critical elements in the education for community participation." They are also of the opinion that health workers should be trained in community-based health care settings in order to develop a thorough understanding of the intricacies of community participation. The need to give serious attention to the training of health care workers in aspects relevant to community participation, is supported by Stewart (1992:19) who maintains that "relevant, progressive curricula are needed to prepare nurses for the challenge of consumer-participation movements". Merely rewriting curricula to accommodate the concept of community participation is relatively simple, but not enough. Practical implementation is more difficult, and must be pursued if effective community participation in health is to be achieved.

To become effective facilitators of community participation, health workers will have to accept certain changes in their roles. They need to become more involved in fostering good community relationships, in educating the community about their rights and responsibilities regarding health, and in promoting community partnership in aspects relevant to health care delivery. The advocacy role of the health worker needs to be developed. All health workers must acquire a thorough understanding of, and appreciation for, human rights to enable them, when necessary, to intervene effectively on behalf of the community in matters affecting their health and well-being.

It is therefore necessary that the training of all health care workers should give adequate attention to the importance of community participation, and the skills necessary to facilitate the process. To enhance community participation, a facilitator must be guided to develop the following:

- belief in the potential of the community
- skill in the participatory approach
- ability to motivate
- ability to create awareness
- understanding of the community culture
- the ability to identify or create structures to assist with the participatory process.

To ensure that the training of health care workers remains appropriate to the needs of the community, there must be ongoing development and regular review of the relevant curricula of health team members. In the process of reviewing the training programmes of health workers, attention should be given to the analysis of training needs on three levels. The three levels involve analysis of the training needs, analysis of syllabuses, and thirdly, analysis of the curriculum as such.

A further aspect to be considered in the evaluation of training programmes concerns the evaluation of the realisation of objectives of a specific programme. On completion of a particular programme, the participating students could be approached to evaluate whether the objectives which had been set for the programme had, in fact, been reached. To do this, the objectives should be clear, both in terms of expected outcomes set by the relevant training institution, and the desired outcomes of the students themselves, and where necessary, subsequent courses should be adapted accordingly.

Educating health workers in the theory and practice of community participation is not only vital to the success of such participation, but is also crucial to the attainment of the objectives of comprehensive primary health care.

4.10 EVALUATION OF COMMUNITY PARTICIPATION

In order to ensure effective, ongoing community participation in health, it is necessary to assess the value of such participation. Bjaras *et al.* (1991:199) suggest an analytical framework, based on the original model of Rifkin *et al.* (1988), to evaluate the degree of change that occurs due to community participation and involvement in health programmes, and maintain that certain (but not all) aspects of the effectiveness of participation can be measured by assessing the occurrence of the following five indicators:

- *needs assessment:* identifying who decides what the needs are, and what is required
- *leadership:* establishing the degree to which the leadership is representative
- *organisation:* identifying the degree of rigidity or flexibility in meeting goals
- *resource mobilisation:* identifying the extent of the human and other resource contributions
- *management:* assessing the degree of involvement of the community in decision-making processes.

Other methods of evaluation of the effectiveness of community participation should also be introduced to assess, *inter alia,* whether the change that occurred is good or not, to identify whether equality in health has, in fact, occurred, and to identify areas still in need of improved community participation. The community must also participate in the process of evaluating its involvement in order to plan future activities more effectively.

4.11 SUMMARY

Communities are becoming increasingly aware of their rights to be involved in decisions that will ultimately affect their health. Factors such as the spiralling cost of medical care, social and political changes and improved standards of education, have all contributed to a greater demand by the community to enter into a partnership with the health team when it comes to matters that affect the community.

The urgency to develop community participation in health can be summarised in the following statement made during the Technical Discussions at the 47th World Health Assembly in Geneva in May 1994:

> "the urgent need for community action for health arises from a combination of factors. On the one hand, the community has gradually come to realize its need and responsibility to assume a greater share of the initiative for its own health care. On the other hand, there has been a growing awareness among health care decision-makers that without community action, much-needed behavioural

changes will not occur and opportunities to prevent major causes of mortality and morbidity will be missed (WHO 1994:8). Community action in health-related matters will, however, not occur automatically."

According to the WHO (1994:34), the success of community action for health initiatives depends on the presence of the following factors:

- a commonality of purpose between all parties concerned
- a sharing of knowledge between the community and the health sector
- the availability of appropriate human and other resources
- joint planning of activities according to commonly agreed upon goals and objectives
- a sensitivity regarding the unique problems experienced by the various parties, as well as the ability to empathise with each other
- political commitment to ensure an active partnership between the community and the formal health sector
- adequate training programmes to enhance leadership development and empowerment of the community, as well as the development of skills in both the health team and the community, necessary to ensure effective partnership.

The importance and inherent value of community participation in health are obvious. Ensuring its effective facilitation and sustainability is more complex. Changing circumstances in South Africa, and acknowledgement of the importance of affirmative action and the right of all people to be part of decision-making processes that affect their health and well-being, highlight the urgency of eliminating all obstacles that could adversely affect the facilitation of community participation in health. Only when all members of the multidisciplinary, intersectoral health team acknowledge the community as an active, equal partner of the team, in a spirit of co-operation and acceptance, will the goal of optimal health for all become more than an unattainable dream.

Bibliography

Alihonou, E., Inoussa, S., Res, L., Sagbohan, M. and Varkevisser, C.M. 1993. *Community participation in primary health care: the case of Gakpe, Benin.* Amsterdam: Royal Tropical Institute (KIT).

ANC policy guidelines on health (health policy forum). 1992. *South African medical journal.* December, Vol. 82:392–3.

Anderson, R.C. 1990. Community cooperation and development. *Sociological practice.* Vol. 8:133–44.

Bernstein, A. and McCarthy, J. 1994. Community organizations in a democratic South Africa. An essay. *Development and democracy. The future of civics?* Vol. 8, November: 68-81

Brearley, S. 1990. *Patient participation: the literature.* Harrow: Scutari Press.

Bopape, M. 1980. Community involvement in community development. *South African journal of sociology.* April, No. 21:31–41.

Bjaras, G., Haglund, B.J.A. and Rifkin, S. 1991. A new approach to community participation assessment. *Health promotion international.* Vol. 6, No. 3:199–206.

Bronwell, B. 1950. *The human community: its philosophy and practice for a time of crisis.* New York: Harper and Brothers Publishers.

Bruyn, S.T. 1963. *Communities in action: pattern and process.* Connecticut: College and University Press.

Chell, E. 1985. *Participation and organisation: a social psychological approach.* London: Macmillan.

Chimere-Dan, G.C. 1996. *Community involvement in urban health programmes.* Johannesburg: International Thomson Publishing (Southern Africa) (Pty) Ltd.

Cooney, C. (Ed.) 1994. *Primary health care - the way to the future.* New York: Prentice-Hall.

Department of Health. 1997. White Paper for the Transformation of the Health System in South Africa. *Government Gazette,* Notice 667 of 1997.

Department of National Health and Population Development. 1991. *Health promotion: information bulletin.* Vol. 1, No. 3. Pretoria: Perskor.

Dreyer, M., Hattingh, S. and Lock, M. 1993. *Fundamental aspects in community health nursing.* Halfway House: Southern.

Farley, S. 1993. The community as partner in primary health care. *Nursing and health care.* May, Vol. 14, No. 5:244–7.

Ferrinho, P. de L.G.M. 1993. Development and health. *CHASA journal of comprehensive health.* April/May, Vol. 4, No. 2:35–8.

Gajanayake, S. and Gajanayake, J. 1993. *Community empowerment: a participatory training manual on community project development.* New York: PACT Publications.

Galaskiewicz, J. 1979. *Exchange networks and community politics.* California: Sage Publications.

Gittell, M. 1980. *Limits to citizen participation: the decline of community organizations.* London: Sage Publications.

IJsselmuiden, C. 1993. The Transvaal School of Public Health: towards education for health. *CHASA journal of comprehensive health.* Vol. 4, Nos. 3 & 4:67-71.

Kramer, R.M. and Specht, H. (Eds) 1983. *Readings in community organization practice.* Englewood Cliffs: Prentice-Hall.

King, L.J. 1996. Community participation in health care delivery: a nursing perspective. DLitt et Phil thesis, University of South Africa.

Mayfield, J.B. 1985. *Go to the people: releasing the rural poor through the people's school system*. Connecticut: Kumarian Press.

Ministry of Health and Social Services (Namibia). 1992. *The official national primary health care/community based health care guidelines*. Windhoek: Government Printer.

National Commission for Higher Education. 1996. *Report: a Framework for Transformation of the Higher Education Sector in South Africa*. Pretoria: NCHE.

Okoro, L.I. 1995. The significance of self help/community participation in health care delivery in South Africa. *CHASA journal of comprehensive health*. September, Vol. 6, No. 3:145-146.

Orem, D.E. 1985. *Nursing: concepts of practice*. 3rd ed. London: Collier Macmillan.

Richards, R.W. 1993. Community partnerships: redirecting health professions education toward primary health care. *Annals of community-oriented education*. Vol. 6:219-229.

Rifkin, S.B. and Cassels, A. 1990. Training managers for primary health care: teaching about community involvement. *Medical teacher*. Vol. 12, No. 1:39–45.

Rifkin, S.B., Muller, F. and Bichmann, W. 1988. Primary health care: on measuring participation. *Social science medicine*. Vol. 26:931–40.

Robb, D., Ferrinho, P. de L.G.M. and Wilson, T.D. 1991. Democracy in health services management. *South African medical journal*. October, Vol. 80:372.

Sekgobela, M.J. 1986. Community participation: the heart of community health. *Nursing RSA Verpleging*. October, Vol. 1, No. 9:30–1.

Shisana, O. and Versfeld, P. 1993. Community participation in health service institutions (issues in medicine). *South African medical journal*. January, Vol. 83:5–8.

Shoo, R. 1991. Training primary health care workers to foster community participation. *World health forum*. Vol. 12:55–62.

Stanhope, M.E. and Lancaster, J. 1992. *Community health nursing: process and practice for promoting health*. 3rd ed. St Louis: Mosby.

Stewart, M.J. 1992. Nursing education as preparation for primary health care partnership with lay persons (news, notes and tips). *Nurse educator*. March/April, Vol. 17, No. 2:8, 15, 19.

Subcommittee: Primary Health Care. 1992. *Strategy for primary health care in South Africa*. Pretoria: Government Printer.

Swanepoel, H.J. and De Beer, F. 1996(a). *Communication for development: a guide for fieldworkers*. Halfway House: International Thomson Publishing.

Swanepoel, H.J. and De Beer, F. 1996(b). *Community capacity building: a guide for fieldworkers and community leaders.* Halfway House: International Thomson Publishing.

Tumwine, J.K. 1989. Community participation as myth or reality: a personal experience from Zimbabwe. *Health policy and planning*. Vol. 4, No. 2:157–61.

Van Rensburg, H.C.J., Fourie, A. and Pretorius, E. 1992. *Health care in South Africa: structure and dynamics*. Pretoria: Academica.

Venter, E.H. 1993. Community participation in health service institutions (letters to the editor). *South African medical journal*. April, Vol. 83:290.

Vroom, V.H. 1960. *Some personality determinants of the effects of participation*. Englewood Cliffs: Prentice-Hall.

Vuori, H. 1984. Overview – community participation in primary health care: a means or an end? *Public health review – IV international congress of the world federation of public health associations*. Vol. 12:331–9.

Wall, T.D. and Lischeron, J.A. 1977. *Worker participation: a critique of the literature and some fresh evidence.* Maidenhead: McGraw-Hill.

Wilson, T.D., Robb, D., Ferrinho, P. de L.G.M. and Ntswanisi, D. 1991. Insights into community participation. *South African medical journal*. October, Vol. 80:372–3.

Woelk, G.B. 1992. Cultural and structural influences in the creation of and participation in community health programmes. *Social science medicine*. Vol. 35, No. 4:419–24.

World Health Organisation. 1974. *Community health nursing: report of a WHO expert committee*. Technical report series No. 558. Geneva: WHO.

World Health Organisation. 1991. *Community involvement in health development*. Technical report series No. 809. Geneva: WHO.

World Health Organisation. 1993. *Community action for health. Report and documentation of the technical discussions of the 46th session of the WHO Regional Committee for South-East Asia.* New Delhi: WHO.

World Health Organisation. 1994(a). *Statements of Dr Hiroshi Nakajima, Director-General, to the Executive Board and the World Health Assembly*. Geneva: WHO

World Health Organisation. 1994(b). *Community action for health*. Background document of the technical discussions. Forty-seventh World Health Assembly. Geneva: WHO.

5

Health promotion: principles and strategies

TRINETTE SWANEPOEL

CHAPTER OBJECTIVES

After reading this chapter, the student should be able to:

- explain the ideology of health promotion
- define health promotion and the empowerment approach
- briefly explain the meaning of the Ottawa Charter of 1986
- explain the principles and policy objectives of the White Paper for the Transformation of the Health System in South Africa
- interpret the transtheoretical model in health promotion
- apply the transtheoretical model of health behaviour change to a health promotion activity
- apply the guidelines for the process of evaluation of workplace health promotion
- implement effective evaluation in health promotion.

5.1 INTRODUCTION

Over the last two decades a growing movement of health professionals, educators, social scientists and community activists has been gathering momentum under the banner of "health promotion". Across the world there are government health promotion strategies, statutory authorities and foundations, professional associations and journals, and consumer interest groups.

While there is by no means unanimity about the so-called "new perspective on health", there is at least a common belief that the reigning "old perspective" on health is too narrow, and that the programmes and institutions designed under its auspices are inadequate responses to the population's interests and health needs. Too much emphasis has been placed on a health care system that is disease-orientated, a so-called "sickness care" system. Caring for people once they have become ill is indeed important, but when resources are marshalled towards this end to the neglect of individual, environmental and biological determinants of health and ill health, priorities need to be examined.

To this extent, health promotion is a reform movement advocating a shift of priorities and resources to align with a broader way of thinking about health, and advocating new and broader social interventions in order to protect, maintain and promote health.

There has recently been confusion in the terminology used to describe health promotion and health education, two separate but interlinked notions. Examining the concept and usage of health promotion, Yeo (1993:226) was tempted to despair that health promotion is the kind of catch-all phrase that means whatever someone wants it to mean. He came across investigators who use the term very broadly to refer to virtually any health-related initiative other than traditional health care, or even encompassing much of traditional health care. Others use the term more restrictively, as referring exclusively to intervention aimed at enabling people to enhance their health. It also appeared that some people use the term synonymously with health education.

The health of a nation is to a certain extent "everybody's business". This is why health promotion brought together people from different disciplines and professions, with different interests and perspectives, to develop and enhance people's health. Health promotion covers those activities that seek to improve the health of communities and individuals. These activities include health education through health education programmes, while others attempt to produce environmental, economic, fiscal, legal and organisational change conducive to good health.

5.2 THE IDEOLOGY OF HEALTH PROMOTION

Health promotion was conceived in the 1970s, born in the 1980s, and matured in the 1990s.

In the 1970s preventable diseases and risk behaviours were primarily tackled through simple education and information (e.g. cancer, heart disease, tobacco). Cattord and St Leger (1996:1-2) call this the first dimension of health promotion. In the 1980s the importance of complementary intervention approaches was emphasised (e.g. the Ottawa Charter's health public policy, community action, personal skills, health services, supportive environments) – the so-called second dimension of health promotion. In the 1990s, the value is learnt of reaching people through the settings where they live and meet (e.g. cities, workplaces, schools, health care settings) – the third dimension of health promotion.

According to Catford and St Leger (1996:2), we need to sustain the momentum and add a fourth dimension to health promotion in the 2000s. This fourth dimension is the most demanding – we need to move. Not just in words but also in actions – from the narrow entry point of disease prevention and control to the wider agenda of health and welfare. The fourth dimension may be mastered if the tried and tested tool kits derived from the first three dimensions are used, together with new approaches, concepts and theories. The challenge now is to respond to the global trends of massive social change which impact on health.

Catford and St Leger (1996:2) mentioned certain social trends that one should be concerned about from a health promotion perspective, of which the seven most important are:

- *Families* – massive shifts in roles, structure and responsibilities
- *Habitats* – increase in urbanisation and rural deprivation
- *Work* – major new patterns, potential and pitfalls
- *Ageing* – progressive lengthening of lifespan and dependency
- *Markets* – sharp movements towards privatisation of services and consumerism
- *Violence* – rising conflicts, victims and refugees
- *Communication* – revolutionary changes in information transfer and learning.

Health promotion built on the work of health education in the 1960s, was considered the driving force behind social change.

Health education was based firmly and deliberately in schools. The view was than only through the process of curriculum innovation, teaching methodologies and pupil-centred learning could education concerned with behavioural change take place. Health promotion offered a radically new concept to the development and enhancement of health. It brought together members of a range of professions and disciplines who realised that there needed to be major changes not only in the way people lived, but also in the conditions under which they lived (MacDonald 1992:71). This corresponds with the view of Yeo (1993:227) that health promotion is interdisciplinary and interprofessional, and different disciplines bring different perspectives and different interests to bear.

In 1977 the World Health Assembly (the central authority for the WHO) resolved that "the main social target of WHO in the coming decades should be the attainment by all citizens of the world by the year 2000 of a level of health that will permit them to lead a socially and economically productive life".

The significant feature of Health for All by the year 2000 (HFA 2000) was the recognition that the main determinants of health lay outside the health sector (water, food, sanitation, housing, employment) and that this implied a global movement in which inequities would be reduced.

The Alma-Ata declaration, recognising primary health care as the key to achieving health for all (HFA), was issued in 1978.

Primary health care, in this original definition, stressed the importance of equity in access to community-based health services that place emphasis on prevention and on action outside the health sector to promote health. Primary health care, according to Alma-Ata, was a comprehensive approach to improving the health status of communities and individuals. Social and economic development was therefore essential to the achievement of health. On the other hand, people themselves do not only have the right, but a duty, to participate individually and collectively in the planning and implementation of their own health care. The Declaration of Alma-Ata made several important assertions which were later to be incorporated into health promotion. Equity was the foundation for achieving HFA 2000.

It was followed in 1984 by a discussion document on concepts and principles for health promotion (WHO 1984).

5.2.1 Health for all

In the Declaration of Alma-Ata (WHO 1978:5) and reaffirmed at Riga (WHO 1988:133), the WHO stressed that the promotion and maintenance of health should become a permanent goal of all nations. An acceptable level of health for all the people of the world can be attained by responding to the challenge to build a national health system based on primary health care.

According to the Director of the WHO Regional Office for Africa (Monekosso 1992:3–5), most developing countries require an appropriate organisational framework for planning and implementing their health development activities. Within such a framework, communities would be encouraged to organise themselves for effective participation in improving their own health and socio-economic status. Monekosso (1992:6) illustrates this statement in a diagram pointing out selected priorities and specific targets for the community, the family and individuals: for operational planning and organisation of health-related activities as well as monitoring and evaluation (Figure 5.1).

As discussed by Joffe and Sutcliffe (1997:169), the health of a population is largely determined by factors outside the jurisdiction of health ministries and health services. Many of the major determinants of health, disease and death are environmental risk factors, not individually chosen aspects of lifestyle. These risk factors may be directly harmful, as in the example of exposure to occupational chemicals. Risk factors may be natural or generated by human activity. The environmental risk factors may also alter people's susceptibility

FIGURE 5.1: A functional breakdown of health for all

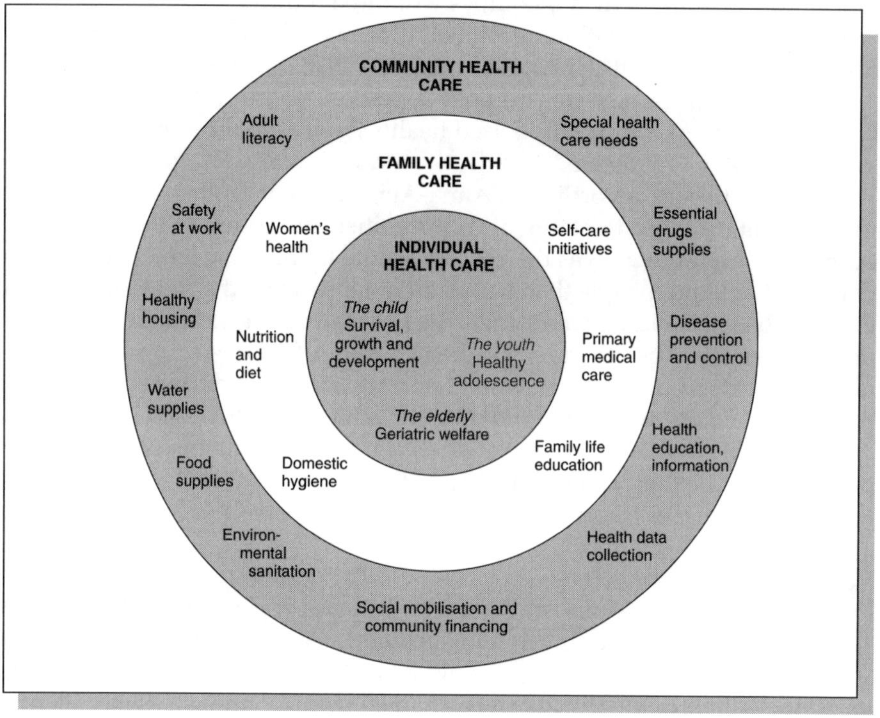

Source: Monekosso (1992:6)

to disease – the availability of sufficient food. In addition, they may operate by making unhealthy choices more likely, for example, the affordability and availability of tobacco or illegal drugs, and also the advertisement of tobacco. It is becoming increasingly clear that one requirement for the promotion of health is that policies in "non-health" areas should take health criteria into account. The need for policy in non-health areas to take account of health has long been emphasised by the WHO, and the need for "intersectoral" collaboration is a key component of its HFA 2000 strategy.

Health promotion should, according to Sindall (1997:6), also promote and lend support to initiatives which may not have an immediate connection with health, but which by their nature are systemic in focus. Action at this level can create more permeable boundaries between different sectors and interests. To make real progress in intersectoral collaboration, there has to be development of the ability to read, interpret and ultimately to shape the context in which collaboration occurs, and not only the development of capacity for working together.

The Department of National Health and Population Development (DNHPD) issued its strategy for the implementation of primary health care in 1992. The strategy is based on the definition of primary health care as stated in the Declaration of Alma-Ata (WHO 1978:5), quoted in a previous chapter.

This implies that people have the right and duty to participate individually and collectively in the planning and implementation of their health care in the spirit of self-determination (WHO 1978:2–3).

The strategy for primary health care (DNHPD 1992:4) underlined the principle that "promotion of health and specific protection of the population is important for sustained economic and social development, and contributes to the quality of life".

As a point of departure, the premise was adopted that in the formulation of the policy guidelines, a future health care system for South Africa would be organised as a unitary structure (DNHPD 1992:1).

This materialised in 1994 when the new Government of National Unity introduced the Reconstruction and Development Programme (RDP) as an integrated, coherent socio-economic policy framework. The political and economic philosophy that underlies the RDP is based on six basic principles (ANC 1994(a):1–7):

- an integrated and sustainable programme
- a people-driven process
- peace and security for all
- nation building
- linking of reconstruction and development
- democratisation of South Africa.

Reconstruction in the health sector will involve a complete transformation of the entire delivery system. This implies that a single, comprehensive, equitable and integrated national health system (NHS) must be created that includes both public and private providers of services and goods. The NHS must be organised at national, provincial, district and community levels.

Recognising this need for total transformation of the health sector in South Africa, the ANC in 1994 initiated a process of developing an overall National Health Plan (NHP) based on the principles and elements of primary health care (PHC). The health of all South Africans will be secured mainly through the achievement of equitable social and economic development. Primary health care will form an integral part of the country's health system and of the overall social and economic development of the community. Central to the PHC approach is full community participation and empowerment, intersectoral collaboration and cost-effective care, as well as integration of health promotion, disease prevention, curative and rehabilitation services (ANC 1994(a):45; ANC 1994(b):9).

In order to help people promote their own health, health practitioners should know the meaning of health.

Health, however, is an extremely difficult concept to define. This is the reason why health is defined in a variety of ways and from different perspectives. It is important for community health practitioners to know what it is that they are promoting.

The first definition of health was issued by the WHO in 1947 (WHO Constitution 1947). It defined health as "a state of complete physical, mental and social well-being, and not merely the absence of disease or infirmity". Health, in this context, is placed in an idealistic sphere, a sphere that is unattainable in everyday life. This definition of health provides no intermediate position or degree of wellness. It deviates from a purely biological orientation (Cookfair 1991:70) and implies a static rather than a dynamic situation. Critics of this definition see health as the ability to adapt continually to constantly changing demands and stimuli.

Nursing theorists have also expressed their views on health. Betty Neuman, one of the foremost health theorists in nursing, created the Neuman system model in which health is equated with a state of wellness, viewed on a continuum.

Health is considered as an open and constantly changing process of experienced energy that ranges along a continuum. The continuum extends from an optimal wellness condition, with available energy at its maximum, to death, which represents total energy depletion.

FIGURE 5.2: The illness/wellness continuum

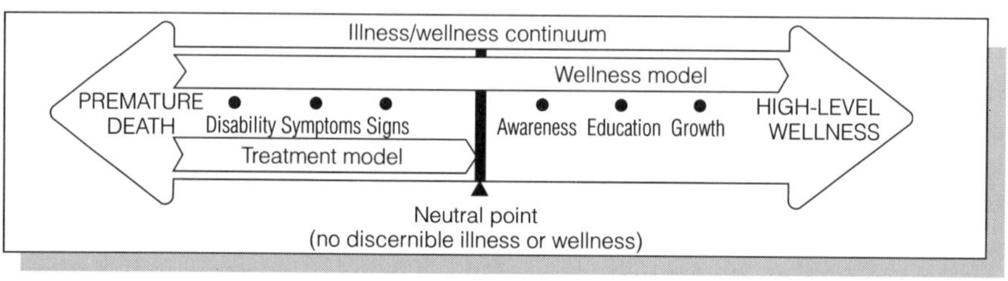

Source: Cookfair (1991:69)

Health, according to Neuman (1989:129), is energy as a result of system balance. The client (community, group, individual) as a system, constantly monitors itself by making adjustments as needed to attain and maintain stability for an optimal state of health. According to Webb (1994:6), it is a recent, popular notion that health and illness are viewed on a continuum. Health can still be achieved despite the existence of a chronic or life-threatening illness, and illness is not inevitable even if certain factors are present within, or impinge upon, humans.

The community health nurse and other health practitioners will benefit from Neuman's system model presenting "health on a continuum" because the client (community, group, individual) can be supported and guided all along the line in any degree of wellness that exists at any given time.

5.2.2 The Ottawa Charter

By the mid-1980s, it was recognised that, if there was to be any significant progress on health for all, some action strategies needed to be developed. This was the purpose of the Ottawa Conference. The Ottawa Charter for Health Promotion which emerged from the first International Conference on Health Promotion held in Ottawa in 1986, could be described as the founding document of health promotion. Health promotion also covers environmental, legal and fiscal measures designed to advance health (WHO 1986:iii).

Five principles underpin this description, which helps incorporate a conceptual framework for health promotion:

- Health promotion involves the population as a whole in the context of their lives rather than focusing on individuals at risk of disease.
- Health promotion targets the determinants of health.
- Health promotion combines diverse but complementary methods.
- Health promotion is aimed at effective community participation.
- Health promotion is basically a health and social activity and not a medical service.

The charter reinforced the commitment of achieving equality in health, but went further in calling for the development of a specific health promotion policy which the charter outlined (WHO 1986).

For the last decade, as explained by Levin and Ziglio (1996:35), the Ottawa Charter for Health Promotion (WHO 1986), has had remarkably wide acceptance as a strategic "checklist" for health promotion. The Charter seems to incorporate elements of traditional concern (personal health skills) with the more recent attention given to community action, the role of health professionals, community supportive resources and healthy public policy. The Charter focuses further on the key functions of enabling, advocacy and mediation.

The Ottawa Charter is a prescription for action, and the five action domains are:

- *Building healthy public policy* – the aim is to ensure safer and health-orientated public services
- *Creating supportive environments* – through health promotion, living and working conditions can be created that are safe and pleasant
- *Developing personal skills* – to help people develop the skills they need to make healthier choices

- *Strengthening community action* – communities must be empowered and have control over their own activities and initiatives
- *Reorienting health services* – the health sector must move beyond the provision of clinical and curative services, to a health promotion approach sensitive to cultural differences.

The Charter's vision of health, its commitment to equity, co-operation and participation, and its interactive means of action, are clearly the way to go. The key to the future is to adopt new health policies with supportive environments as their goal and healthy public policy as their principal instrument.

The Ottawa Charter (WHO 1986) considered the pivotal role of a "healthy public policy" to be the key requirement for avoiding unnecessary disease and the achievement of a socially and economically productive life.

The view of the WHO concerning health promotion is accepted worldwide. It was accepted by the Republic of South Africa in 1990, when the government committed itself to the rendering of primary health care.

5.3 WHAT IS HEALTH PROMOTION?

Health promotion may be defined as the process of enabling people (individuals and communities) to increase control over the determinants of health, and thereby improve it. Health education is a central tool in this process. Health education is part of, but not the sum of, health promotion. This indicates that health promotion and health education cannot be referred to as one and the same.

The WHO (1987:12) views health promotion as a "unifying concept for those who recognise the need for change in the ways and conditions of living, in order to promote health". The major strategy for achieving the global target of health for all by the year 2000 is considered by the WHO to be the health promotion programme. Health promotion in this sense is concerned with all the factors which influence health. According to Tone, Tilford and Robinson (1990:3), they recognised four major influences that affect health status:

- health and medical services
- genetic endowment
- individual behaviours
- socio-economic and physical environment.

Health is therefore viewed as both a positive state of well-being and an absence of disease.

In addition to the principle that health is more than the absence of disease but rather a state of physical, mental and social well-being, the new health promotion programme of the WHO (1987) differs from earlier concerns in the following important ways:

- Health promotion is acknowledged as an intersectoral activity. Following the tenets of primary health care (WHO 1978), health promotion is not considered to be the preserve of the medical services. The professions, industry and trade unions should assume the responsibility to ensure that the prerequisites for health lie outside the health sector.
- The programme asserts the importance of the socio-economic and physical environment in determining health and illness. As indicated in the Ottawa Charter for Health Promotion (1986), the WHO is concerned to "build healthy public policy" and "create supportive environments".
- The programme argues that health and medical services must be reorientated in order to meet consumer needs in a responsive and holistic way. This process should increase community participation and lay involvement. People must be helped to gain control over their own health.

Catford and Nutbeam gave the following explanation for health promotion in 1984:

> "Health promotion seeks to improve or protect health through behavioural, socio-economic, biological and environmental changes. It embraces the concepts of disease prevention as well as the notion of positive health – the promotion of or sense of physical and mental well-being. A major emphasis is to make the healthy choices, the easy choices. Health education is a core component and it is unlikely that health promotion will succeed without it."

The above definition of health promotion indicates a philosophical basis of self-empowerment. The centrepiece of the charter is the concept of "enabling", which integrates health and freedom and the individual and the community.

One of the virtues of the concept of enabling as articulated in the charter, according to Yeo (1993:233), is that it regards freedom and responsibility not as a given but as a task, something that has to be developed and nurtured. Enabling is based on the idea that in order to realise freedom and assume greater responsibility for their health, individuals may require help in the form of know-how, resources and power to assume greater control.

A related virtue of the charter concept of enabling is that it bridges rather than divides the individual and the community. Responsibility is attributed not simply to individuals, but to communities, or the individual in the community – in a family, in a neighbourhood, in a workplace or in a support group. The target of health promotion is not so much the imprudent and community-threatening individual, as it is communities – or individuals in community – lacking the know-how, control and resources "to achieve their fullest health potential". The goal of health promotion along these lines is "full and organised community participation and ultimate self-reliance, with individuals, families and communities assuming more responsibility for their own health"(WHO 1978:153).

The charter recognises that community focus is important, not only because supportive and effective communities are beneficial for individual health, but also because the solutions to many health problems, such as an unsafe workplace or stress, require co-operative and collective action.

From this perspective it is clear that at the core of health promotion is personal empowerment and communal action. Therefore the success of any health promotion strategy, for example to reduce at-risk (unprotected) sexual behaviour and increase AIDS/HIV-related information, can ultimately be measured by its ability to foster and sustain personal empowerment and communal action. Empowerment should be the primary goal and guiding value of health promotion (Livingstone 1993:191).

5.3.1 Empowerment approach

Fahlberg, as quoted by Williams (1995:37), proposed a definition of empowerment that includes the development of the capacities of both the community and the individual to enhance their own health, and the removal of structural and social barriers, such as poverty, which inhibit the attainment of health. From this perspective, an empowerment approach in health promotion involves the elements of facilitating the process of individual growth and development, and a commitment to challenging injustice.

An approach to health promotion that recognises the rights of communities and individuals to identify their own health needs, to make their own choices and to take action to achieve them, is describe by Williams (1995:38) as an "empowerment" approach. This empowerment approach rejects the individualistic values that have so strongly influenced health promotion practices, ceasing to define problems in terms of apathy, personal ignorance and incompetence, and to see "solutions" in terms of lifestyle changes. In contrast, the empowerment approach focuses on realising the potential for growth and development of people as communities and individuals, and on removing the structural barriers of gender, race, class, age and physical ability that inhibit these.

An empowerment approach to health promotion challenges the traditional medical model in which the health professional, as expert in possession of specialist knowledge, prescribes what the community and individuals need to know, passes on that information and expects compliance. If health promotion professionals are to understand and espouse an empowerment approach in their work, they need opportunities to explore the process of empowerment in their own professional training and development.

According to Williams (1995:37), an empowerment approach offers a means whereby health promotion professionals can raise awareness of health inequalities and of the underlying sociopolitical causes of ill health, and facilitate social and political change to promote health.

Supporters of the empowerment approach such as Abel, Boland, Durand, Geolot, Goodson, Isham and Steele (1995:75-83), agree that this approach to health promotion is based on the view that health professionals assist communities or at-risk aggregates in identifying their own needs, priorities, problems and solutions.

5.3.2 Health promotion activities

Health promotion is often referred to as an "umbrella" term, encompassing a range of activities. This view is clarified by Ewles and Simnett (1992:22), who provide a framework for classifying health promotion activities. In Figure 5.3 those activities which aim to improve people's health are mapped out.

It is important to notice that this framework consists of nine categories, divided between two sets of activities. The first set of activities comprises two activities, illness and disability services, i.e. providing personal social services and health care services for the ill and disabled. The second set comprises seven types of positive health activities which are personal, social and environmental changes aiming to prevent ill health and develop healthier living conditions and ways of life. These two sets of activities overlap because they are often closely related in practice, and they both contribute towards promoting better health (Ewles and Simnett 1992.21–2).

5.4 WHITE PAPER FOR THE TRANSFORMATION OF THE HEALTH SYSTEM IN SOUTH AFRICA

In 1997, the White Paper for the transformation of the health system in South Africa was published by the Ministry of Health. The object of the White Paper is to present to the people of South Africa a set of principles and policy objectives upon which the Unified National Health System of South Africa will be based.

Poverty, poor physical and social conditions, such as lack of adequate access to safe water, poor housing and sanitation, have impacted negatively on the health status of a large proportion of the population of South Africa. Health programmes have been disease-focused and based on theoretical frameworks that were not always sympathetic to community perspectives. The transition to democracy, reconstruction and development and the

FIGURE 5.3: Health promotion: activities for better health

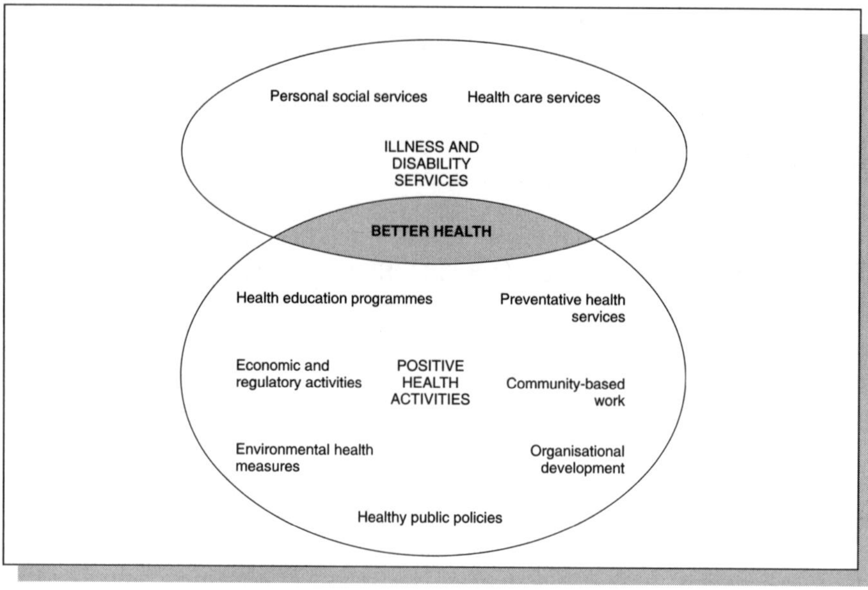

Source: Ewles and Simnett (1992:2)

principles elaborated by the RDP (ANC 1994), are important cornerstones for developing necessary health promotion initiatives.

The aim of health promotion in South Africa is to improve the health of all its citizens through creating a physical, social, economic and political environment which helps to make healthy choices easy choices (RSA 1997:178).

Areas of principal activity for an effective health promotion strategy which are outlined in the White Paper, are the development of public policies, promoting healthy physical and social environments, skills development, community action and empowerment of communities and individuals to promote their own health, and a focused reorientation of the health services.

The following objectives are formulated:

- to promote and develop health promotion activity in government and civil society
- to develop a skilled cadre of health promoters
- to contribute to the development and achievement of a healthy nation.

Health promotion will be established as an integral part of the National Health System, and developed in accordance with the principles which underpin the WHO movement "Health for all by the year 2000".

- *Equity* – similar opportunities with regard to health for everyone
- *Empowerment and respect* – health promotion activities should be designed to increase and enhance the control that communities and individuals have over their own health
- *Participation* – communities and individuals will be involved as respected partners in the planning and implementation of health promotion programmes
- *Intersectoral activity* – multidisciplinary and intersectoral collaboration wherever relevant and possible
- *Standards of practice* – encouragement of highest standards of practice, based upon researched needs and adequate evaluation.

Partnership will be established with all stakeholders, especially with communities, to work towards achieving a nationwide impact on the major health problems, and to achieve optimum health for the nation as a whole.

The scope of health promotion activity will be in accordance with the five "action domains" outlined by the Ottawa Charter:

- Promoting public health policy in all sectors of South African society, e.g. fluoridation of water supplies
- Creating supportive environments, i.e. ensuring that the South African environment (social and physical) is healthy and that healthy behaviour is promoted, e.g. by the creation of smoke-free environments
- Developing personal skills in the formal and informal education sectors, e.g. by the provision of basic health care
- Supporting community action by facilitating and encouraging communities to take action that will improve their health and resolve problems
- Reorienting health care to provide services which are relevant, appropriate and close to where the people live (RSA 1997:178–183).

5.5 THEORY IN HEALTH PROMOTION

5.5.1 Overview

It is often asserted that health promotion is based in experience and that the field of health promotion is barren of theoretical perspectives. Dean and McQueen (1996:7) hold the view that at the heart of this assertion is the perceived lack of any sound theoretical foundation purporting to explain health-related behaviours.

Health promotion evolved out of an action-orientated practice field, using knowledge derived from research conducted in other disciplines. Many disciplines have the necessary knowledge for understanding health promotion. When there is relevant and valid knowledge available for programme development, prioritising implementation can contribute to effective health promotion action. A strategy for theory construction is to move to a multidisciplinary approach. A sound knowledge base for action is thus a prerequisite for achieving health promotion policy and practice. Dean and McQueen (1996:7) argue further that, while there is debate on the relevant importance of theory in health promotion, there is agreement that the focus of public health needs to be on health rather than on disease. This means that the focus of the theoretical perspectives in health promotion, which still largely stem from a medical model of disease, needs to shift towards the survivors of adversity, rather than those who succumbed to disease.

A consensus view seems to be developing that health promotion theories need to be contextual and dynamic in order to guide research that improves knowledge about the real complex causal processes affecting health in communities. Only health promotion theories that build in the interacting casual influences operating in the daily lives of human beings, can avoid misdirected health promotion policy and programme implementation (Dean and McQueen 1996:7-9).

5.5.2 Theory in health behaviour

The basic components of a theory for health-related behaviour, and by analogy health promotion, should, according to McQueen (1996:29), derive from the research base of this century's work in the behavioural and social sciences. McQueen (1996:32) mentioned four reasons for the importance of theory building in any field of human endeavour, and in particular the field of health promotion:

- Theory provides the guiding light for what to study (and what not to study)
- Theory serves the useful function of defining whatever we cannot understand
- A theoretical perspective helps to understand how different pieces fit together and why some combinations of variables would be valued more than others
- Adopting a theoretical approach helps define the appropriate methods.

The basic components of a theory of health-related behaviour is that it is dynamic; it focuses on change and movement rather than stability. Changes are, however, significant departures from the usual behavioural patterns. The theoretical challenge is to explain how and when these changes occur. Any behaviour has a prevalence; change in behaviour has an incidence, but one cannot have a prevalence of change.

Change in behaviour is chiefly characterised by the taking up, alteration or cessation of a given behaviour over some defined period of time. What seems clear is that any theory of behavioural change must account for these types of change, but that over the lifespan, different causal factors and determinants of change may operate. Initiating a behaviour involves a different mixture of individual, biological and social components to cessation, and that in turn, the next taking up of the behaviour of a cessation will involve yet another multifactorial mixture. Behaviour takes place within a context, meaning within a combination of social and environmental factors. Behaviours are at different levels. Some behaviours are very fundamental while others seem very trivial from the individual's perspective. Time is a fundamental component in behaviour and behaviour change. Changes in behaviour often occur at specified points of time. Both individual and population behaviours vary over time. Viewed over time, behaviours occur over a continuum from continuous to once in a lifespan. Each and every behaviour has its own dimension of time (McQueen 1996:29-30).

5.5.3 The transtheoretical model of health behaviour change

The transtheoretical model has been developed by Dr J Prochaska and his colleagues over the last several decades. This model uses a temporal dimension, the stages of change, to integrate processes and principles of change from different theories of intervention, hence the name "transtheoretical". Stages of change is the central organising construct of this model. The model posits that health behaviour change involves progress through six stages of change. Ten processes of change have been identified for producing progress along with a set of intervening or dependent measures.

Prochaska and Velicer (1997:6) point out that the transtheoretical model provides an innovative approach to health promotion that emphasises:

- behaviour change viewed as a progression through a series of stages (precontemplation, contemplation, preparation, action, maintenance)
- matching the most relevant independent variables and the most appropriate dependent variables to particular stages of change
- designing health promotion interventions that meet the needs of the individual at each stage of change
- maximising impact on entire population at risk (by employing practice recruitment and stage-matched, interactive and individualised interventions)
- emphasising the importance of integrating health promotion programmes across multiple channels (e.g. homes, communities, workplace).

(a) Stages of change

The stage construct of the transtheoretical model is important in part because it represents a temporal dimension. This model constructs change as a process involving progress through a series of six stages:

- **Stage 1:** Precontemplation
  In this stage people are not intending to take action in the foreseeable future, usually measured as the next six months. People may be in this stage because they are underinformed or uninformed about the consequences of their behaviour. People may have tried to change this behaviour a number of times and become demoralised about their ability to change. Both groups of people tend to avoid talking, reading or thinking about their high-risk behaviours. The fact is that traditional health promotion programmes were not ready for such individuals and were not motivated to match their needs.
- **Stage 2:** Contemplation
  This is the stage in which people are intending to change in the next six months. People are more aware of the pros of changing but are also acutely aware of the cons.
- **Stage 3:** Preparation
  In this stage, people are intending to take action in the immediate future, usually measured as the next six months. These individuals have a plan of action, such as joining a health education class or relying on a self-change approach. These are the people that should be recruited for such action-oriented programmes as exercise or weight loss.
- **Stage 4:** Action
  In this stage, people have made specific overt modifications in their lifestyles within the past six months. Since action is observable, behaviour change has often been equated with action. People must attain a criterion that health promotion practitioners agree is sufficient to reduce risks for disease.
- **Stage 5:** Maintenance
  In this stage of maintenance, people are working to prevent relapse but they do not apply change processes as frequently as individuals in action. Relapse is one form of regression, which is a return to an earlier stage. Relapse is the return from action or maintenance to an earlier stage.
- **Stage 6:** Termination
  Termination is the stage in which people have zero temptation and one hundred per cent self-efficacy. No matter whether these individuals are depressed, lonely or stressed, they are sure they will not return to their old unhealthy habit as a way of coping. It is as if these people never acquired that habit in the first place.

(b) Processes of change

Processes of change are the overt and covert activities that people use to progress through the stages. Processes of change provide important guides for intervention programmes.

- *Consciousness raising* – involves increased awareness about the causes, consequences and cures for a particular problem behaviour. Feedback, education, confrontation and media campaigns are interventions that can increase awareness.
- *Dramatic relief* – initially produces increased emotional experiences followed by reduced effect if appropriate action can be taken. Personal testimonies, grieving, role-playing and media campaigns are examples of techniques that can move people emotionally.
- *Self-re-evaluation* – combines both cognitive and affective assessment of one's self-image with and without a particular unhealthy habit, such as one's image as an active person. Healthy role-models, value clarification and imagery are techniques that can move individuals to re-evaluate themselves.
- *Environmental re-evaluation* – combines both affective and cognitive assessments of how the presence or asence of a personal habit affects one's social environment, such as the effect of smoking on others. Family interventions, documentaries and empathy training can lead to such reassessments.
- *Self-liberation* – is both the belief that one can change and the commitment and recommitment to act on that belief. Public testimonies, New Year's resolutions, and multiple rather than single choices can enhance self-liberation (willpower).
- *Social liberation* – requires an increase in social opportunities or alternatives especially for individuals who are relatively oppressed or deprived. Empowerment procedures, advocacy and appropriate policies can produce increased opportunities for minority health promotion, and can also be used to help all people change, such as having smoke-free zones.
- *Counter-conditioning* – requires the learning of healthier behaviours that can substitute for problem behaviours. Assertion can counter peer pressure and relaxation can counter stress.
- *Stimulus control* – removes cues for unhealthy habits and adds prompts for healthier alternatives. Self-help groups, avoidance and environmental re-engineering can provide stimuli that support change and reduce risks for relapse (planning parking lots with a 2-minute walk to the nearest office).
- *Contingency management* – provides consequences for taking steps in a particular direction. Reinforcements are emphasised, since a philosophy of the stage model of health behaviour change, is to work in harmony with the way in which people change naturally. Overt and covert reinforce-

ments, positive self-statements and group recognition are procedures for increasing reinforcement and the probability that healthier responses will be repeated.
- *Helping relationships* – combine trust, caring and acceptance, as well as support for the healthy behaviour change. A therapeutic alliance, counsellor calls and buddy systems can be sources of social support.

(c) Intervening measures

The transtheoretical model of health behaviour change also includes a set of intervening or dependent measures such as the pros and cons from the decisional balance, self-efficacy and temptation.
- *Decisional balance.* Decisional balance reflects people's relative weighing of the pros and cons of changing.
- *Self-efficacy.* Self-efficacy is the situation-specific confidence individuals have that they can cope with high-risk situations without relapsing to their high-risk or unhealthy habit.
- *Temptation.* Temptation reflects the intensity of urges to engage in a specific habit when in the midst of difficult situations. Emotional distress, craving and positive social situations are three factors reflecting the most common types of tempting situations.

In addition to the research undertaken by Prochaska and Velicer (1997:38-40) on the transtheoretical model of health behaviour change, McQueen (1996:31) argues that basically health behaviour change depends largely on the following three factors:
- characteristics of the population or individual with the potential to change
- characteristics of the behaviour itself
- characteristics of the social environmental context of the behaviour.

The transtheoretical model of health behaviour change, as described by Prochaska and Velicer (1997:387-40) has concentrated on six stages of change, ten processes of change and the pros and cons of changing, self-efficacy and temptation.

5.6 WORKPLACE HEALTH PROMOTION

There has been considerable interest in the workplace as a setting for health promotion in western countries but also in South Africa. It has been argued that there are economic incentives for employers to take part in health promotion, since it can reduce absenteeism and health costs. Workplace health promotion can reach a large segment of the population, particularly young men, who are difficult to target through other access points.

Health promotion activity in the workplace has been increasing in recent years as companies have become more aware of economic advantages of investing in the health of their employees. Large companies are the most likely to engage in health promotion activities, but public sector organisations are more likely to have health promotion programmes. In South Africa, the National Health Plan (NHPSA) initiated by the African National Congress (ANC), states that it is the responsibility of the state to create a framework within which health is promoted. Priority programmes have been developed which will include the development of programmes for occupational health. In addition, the health priorities will also include health promotion, environmental health and combating substance abuse. In all health programmes and activities a special emphasis will be given to health promotion (ANC 1994(a):11).

Workplace health promotion programmes have the potential to be effective since they can readily foster social pressure for behaviour change and introduce incentives for healthy behaviour. Health promotion in the workplace offers the opportunity to modify the structural environment by modifying workplace hazards or encouraging the canteen to offer more healthy food choices (Xing Fa, Xueqi, Wan Qing and Redman 1995:25).

Workplaces could be responsible for many aspects of the health of their employees, such as being responsible for providing food, health care, child care, support during retirement and accommodation. Workplaces frequently provide leisure activities, including social recreation and sport. This means that workplace health promotion can effectively address many aspects of the individual's life and environment. The range of health promotion activities varies enormously and may include programmes for prevention and control of risks at work, general health assessments, assessment of fitness for work after injury, smoking cessation programmes, promotion of exercise and healthy nutrition, and the promotion of the psychological well-being of the worker (Springett and Dugdill 1995:89; ANC 1994(a):46).

Springett and Dugdill (1995:89) came to the conclusion that despite the encouraging development in health promotion activities, the emphasis has been on changing the individual's lifestyle. In South Africa's policy on health promotion as introduced in the National Health Plan (ANC 1994(a):41) and the Reconstruction and Development Programme (RDP) (ANC 1994(b):47), the democratic government of South Africa committed itself to ensure that all South African citizens have the right to a decent quality of life, through:

- equitable access to natural resources
- safe and healthy living and working environments
- a participatory decision-making process around environmental issues, empowering communities to manage their natural environment (ANC 1994(b):39).

Health promotion and health protection of the worker will be integrated into the national strategies for health development. Occupational health services and programmes "will emphasise a comprehensive, multidisciplinary and participatory approach, stressing both prevention and rehabilitation, and identifying high-risk and underserved occupational groups" (ANC 1994(a):49).

The RDP (ANC 1994(b):47) aims to promote mental health by implementing comprehensive strategies to change behaviour. These strategies include education programmes, reduction of advertising and an increase in the price of alcohol and tobacco. Health promotion programmes will be set up with primary responsibility for national level mass media campaigns (ANC 1994(a):41).

Although it may become increasingly easy to persuade companies to invest in health promotion, it has proved to be more difficult to persuade employers to implement relevant health promotion programmes in the appropriate way, and to evaluate them properly.

Evaluation of workplace health promotion activity has predominantly focused on the measurement of health behaviour change, such as measuring the reduction in the number of smokers immediately after an anti-smoking campaign, or measuring body weight after a fitness programme. The wider issues of benefits to a company from engaging in health promotion programmes, as well as looking at the health impact of organisational change such as workplace restructuring (e.g. changes to working time and new job designs), according to Springett and Dugdill (1995:90), present greater challenges to the workplace health agenda for the year 2000.

The most successful health promotion programmes are those in which:

- employers and employees participate actively in deciding what programmes to introduce and how to implement them
- the aims and objectives are clear
- evaluation is an integral part of the programme planning and implementation process.

5.6.1 Evaluation principles

Whatever health promotion programme is planned, there are certain basic principles that need to be followed to achieve effective programme evaluation:

- *Participation.* Participation is a primary requisite for programme evaluation. The process of health promotion programme evaluation should be a participatory one. An evaluation should show all the perspectives of different interest groups, especially those of the less dominant ones (both management and workforce). It is true that people have different perceptions of what an programme evaluation should entail. Their views will vary according to context, depending on organisational structures and priorities. It is therefore important to tell people what the health promotion programme includes. If workers are involved, their mental health status may be enhanced and intervention strategies adhered to. Workplaces have different cultural values and so do groups within them.

- *Clarity of purpose.* Clarity of the purpose of the evaluation of the health promotion programme is another key requisite, and involves the following evaluation measures:

  Process evaluation – measures what actually occurs during the planning and implementation of a certain health promotion programme.

  Impact evaluation – looks at the immediate effects of a health promotion programme, for example improved reported health status, and

  Outcome evaluation – measures long-term effects such as the reduction in sickness absenteeism over a five-year period.

  Ideally, a balance of process, impact and outcome evaluation is required in order to assess progress towards planned health promotion goals, as well as to be able to understand what health promotion activities are successful and why they are successful.
- *Timing.* To ensure that relevant data are collected throughout the duration of programme evaluation, it is important that decisions about evaluation are taken at the same time as workplace health promotion activities are being planned.
- *Relevant data.* The types of information collected will also depend on who the evaluation is for. Information can be collected at different levels. At the level of the individual, regular fitness testing provides workers with feedback on how well they are doing during participation in a health promotion activity intervention. This encourages further information. At group level, a questionnaire will provide information on change in behaviours, attitudes and beliefs before, during and after a programme. At company level, data on absenteeism rates will provide information on how well the programme is doing and whether continued investment is worthwhile. Timing of information collection is crucial for measuring evaluation effectiveness.
- *Sensitivity.* The collection of information raises sensitive and often disturbing ethical issues. If workers perceive that the information will be used to decide who will be made redundant, their co-operation is likely to be limited and the data unreliable. Problems are most likely to be resolved if the evaluation process has been a participatory process.

TABLE 5.1: Guidelines for the process of evaluation of workplace health promotion

Steps	Main actions	Associated actions
Step 1	Clarify aims and objectives of the proposed health promotion programme	Get people on board Set up an evaluation group Check out what the real health problem is Establish baseline information
Step 2	Design the framework for evaluation and decide what questions will be asked	Decide what the purpose of the evaluation is and who is going to use the information Decide what useful questions to ask in relation to achieving aims and objectives Decide from whom to collect the information Decide on process and/or outcome evaluation
Step 3	Design the framework for evaluation and decide how to measure change	Decide what to measure and which methods to use Decide on target population Decide when to collect the information
Step 4	Collect the data	Make sure data collection does not add to people's workload and is unobtrusive Make sure people are still on board Keep people informed by regular feedback
Step 5	Evaluate the results to determine effectiveness of the programme	Interpret data in association with evaluation group Compare what actually happened with what is expected
Step 6	Make recommendations	Clarify what is useful Cover practical changes for immediate implementation Include the costs and benefits of not implementing Challenge existing beliefs Look at long-term changes that may not yet be visible

Source: Springett and Dugdill (1995:93)

5.6.2 Evaluation process

To encourage employers to adopt effective health promotion programmes and practices and to evaluate them, Springett and Dugdill (1995:92-94), described six main steps for an effective process of evaluation. These steps are outlined as guidelines for the process of evaluation of workplace health promotion in Table 5.1.

The basic premise of the guidelines (Table 5.1) is that the purpose of evaluation is to provide useful information in the most practical way possible. Evaluation is a learning process which forms an integral part of action for change in the workplace, and should therefore not be done in isolation but be part of an integrated approach to problem analysis, planning and implementation.

Although the guidelines for the process of evaluation of workplace health promotion do not offer a definite answer to all evaluation problems, by following the stages in the guidelines, there will be greater clarity among all the participants about the benefits and the validity and reliability of the information gathered.

5.6.3 Barriers to effective evaluation

Health promotion should be holistic, involving interventions which focus both on people and on the environment, using multiple strategies to achieve its end. A strategy may be seen as a theory of how to achieve a goal, based on assumptions about reality relationships. The barriers to achieving this are also barriers which prevent effective evaluation.

Traditions of occupational health practices to which most workplace activities have been confined, are based on practice and knowledge that evolved within the context of health and safety legislation, and are divorced from wider public health issues. Springett and Dugdill (1995:90-92) are further of the opinion that workplace health promotion has tended to focus on health screening and the assessment and control of threats to workplace health that arise from the physical, biological and chemical environments. Such approaches have failed to take into account newly recognised threats to health, particularly due to the psychosocial environment.

Occupational health professionals are mostly from single-discipline backgrounds and may be unfamiliar with the multidisciplinary participatory approach that health promotion demands, and which could challenge current professional practice. As a result there has been resistance to a broader approach.

Another barrier to effective evaluation lies in the area of health promotion itself. One reason why evaluation has been neglected in the past is that it tended to be viewed somewhat negatively by those involved in health promotion.

The field of operation of workplace health promotion is potentially wider than the workplace itself. It cannot disputed that work has a major influence on the general well-being of the workforce, and health promotion activities in the workplace can artificially separate work from other aspects of people's lives, particularly in the case of women. Women suffer increasing stress from the demands of multiple roles, such as being a wife and mother, a worker and a provider of care for elderly relatives.

This lack of attention to different groups' specific needs is also reflected in the way needs assessment is undertaken. It is now seen as good health promotion practice to undertake a health needs assessment before determining the nature of an intervention. Conventional approaches to health needs assessment tend to reinforce existing practice. Mechanisms need to be in place to allow different experiences to be incorporated and articulated in the agenda of change, if workers' realities differ from those of management or health professionals.

Lack of resources - human, financial and time - is a major barrier to effective evaluation in health promotion. A lack of resources is a particular problem with medium-sized and small enterprises. This is often also the case among larger organisations, except where there are well-developed health policies, specific health budgets and strong traditions and philosophies of human resource management.

The effectiveness of evaluation in health promotion depends on the way it is undertaken. There should be clarity as to the purpose of the evaluation, since the type of evaluation depends on its purpose (Springett and Dugdill 1995:88-98).

5.7 SUMMARY

In this chapter the ideology of health promotion is explained as background to a concept that was born in the 1980s and matured in the 1990s. The view of the WHO, as outlined in the Ottawa Charter on health promotion, is linked to the South African situation. The strategy for the implementation of primary health care in South Africa was compiled in 1992 and followed by the Reconstruction and Development Programme and National Health Plan in 1994. The whole national health system of South Africa will be driven by the primary health care approach.

Health promotion is changing in a rapidly changing world. Health promotion is reinventing itself, now following the shifting contours of social, economic and political change, and changes in public preferences and expectations.

An empowerment approach in health promotion involves the elements of facilitating the process of individual growth and development and a commitment to challenging injustice.

The White Paper for the transformation of the health system in South Africa emphasises that the aim of health promotion is to improve the health of all South African citizens through creating a physical, social, economic and political environment which helps to make it easier for people to make healthy choices.

This chapter includes an explanation by Prochaska and Velicer on their transtheoretical model of health behaviour change. This model consists of six stages of change, and ten processes of change for producing progress along with decisional balance, self-efficacy and zero temptation.

Evaluation of health activity in the workplace is part of the process of quality assurance. If the process is initiated correctly, then it becomes a natural and automatic review activity, integral to the whole programme of health activity and work tasks.

Evaluation is about measuring change, and the ultimate success of an evaluation depends on the uses to which it is put by management.

The effectiveness of evaluation in health promotion depends on the way it is undertaken. There should be clarity as to the purpose of the evaluation, since the type of evaluation depends on its purpose (Springett and Dugdill 1995:88-98).

Bibliography

Abel, E., Boland, M., Durand, B., Geolot, D., Goodson, J., Isham, G. and Steele, L. 1995. Workforce and community health care needs: a model to link service, education, and the community. *Family community health.* Vol. 18, No. 2:75–79.

African National Congress. 1994(a). *A national health plan for South Africa.* Maseru: Bähr Mapping and Printing.

African National Congress. 1994(b). *The reconstruction and development programme.* Johannesburg: Umanyano.

Catford, J. and Nutbeam, D. 1984. Towards a definition of health education and health promotion. *Health education journal.* Vol. 43, Nos. 2&3:1.

Catford, J. and St Leger, L. 1996. Moving into the next decade – and a new dimension. *Health promotion international.* Vol. 11, No. 1:1–3.

Cookfair, J.M. 1991. *Nursing process and the practice in the community.* St Louis: Mosby.

Dean, K. and McQueen, D. 1996. Theory in health promotion: introduction. *Health promotion international.* Vol. 11, No. 1:7–9.

Department of National Health and Population Development. 1992. *Strategy for primary health care in South Africa.* Pretoria.

Ewles, L. and Simnett, I. 1992. *Promoting health: a practical guide.* 2nd ed. London: Scutari Press.

Joffe, M. and Sutcliffe, J. 1997. Developing policies for a healthy environment. *Health promotion international.* Vol. 12, No. 2:169–173.

Levin, L.S. and Ziglio, E. 1996. Health promotion as an investment strategy: considerations on theory and practice. *Health promotion international.* Vol. 11, No. 1:33–40.

Livingstone, I.L. 1993. HIV/AIDS control in Africa: the importance of epidemiological and health approaches. *Health promotion international.* Vol. 8, No. 3:187–97.

MacDonald, G. 1992. Health promotion and sustainable development. *Health promotion international.* Vol. 7, No. 2:71–2.

McQueen, D. 1996. The search for theory in health behaviour and health promotion. *Health promotion international.* Vol. 1, No. 1:27–32.

Monekosso, G.L. 1992. An organisational framework for achieving health for all in developing countries. *International journal of health planning and management.* Vol. 1, No. 7:3–22.

Neuman, B. 1989. *The Neuman systems model.* Norwalk: Appleton and Lange.

Prochaska, J. and Velicer, W. 1997. The transtheoretical model of health behaviour change. *American journal of health promotion.* Vol. 12, No. 1:6, 38–47.

Republic of South Africa. 1997. White Paper for the transformation of the Health System in South Africa. *Government Gazette.* 382, (17910): 178–183.

Sindall, C. 1997. Intersectoral collaboration: the best of times, the worst of times. *Health promotion international.* Vol. 12, No. 1:5–7.

Springett, J. and Dugdill, L. 1995. Workplace health promotion programmes: towards a framework for evaluation. *Health education journal.* Vol. 54:88–98.

Stanhope, M.E. and Lancaster, J. 1992. *Community health nursing: process and practice for promoting health.* St Louis: Mosby.

Tone, K., Tilford, S. and Robinson, Y. 1990. *Health education: effectiveness and efficiency.* London: Chapman and Hall.

Webb, P. 1994. *Health promotion and patient education.* London: Chapman and Hall.

Williams, J. 1995. Education for empowerment: implications for professional development and training in health promotion. *Health education journal.* Vol. 54:37–47.

Wilson-Barnett, J. and Clark, J.M. 1993. *Research in health promotion and nursing.* London: Macmillan.

World Health Organisation. 1947. *Chronicle of the WHO.* Vol. 1, No. 3:1.

World Health Organisation. 1978. *Primary health care. Report of the international conference on primary health care.* Alma-Ata, USSR. 6–12 September 1978. Geneva.

World Health Organisation. 1984. *Health promotion: a discussion document on the concepts and principles.* Copenhagen: WHO Regional Office for Europe.

World Health Organisation. 1986. *Ottawa charter for health promotion: an international conference on health promotion.* November 17–21. Copenhagen: WHO Regional Office for Europe.

World Health Organisation. 1987. *Health promotion: concepts and principles in action, a policy framework*. Copenhagen: WHO Regional Office for Europe.

World Health Organisation. 1988. *From Alma-Ata to the year 2000: reflections at the midpoint*. Geneva: WHO.

Xing Fa, G., Xueqi, G., Wan Qing, Z. and Redman, S. 1995. Workplace health promotion in Shanghai: needs assessment in four different industries. *Health promotion international*. Vol. 10, No. 1:25–32.

Yeo, M. 1993. Towards an ethic of empowerment for health promotion. *Health promotion international*. Vol. 8, No. 3:225–35.

6

Communication in health care delivery

TRINETTE SWANEPOEL

CHAPTER OBJECTIVES

After reading this chapter, the student should be able to:

- discuss the basic components of the communication process
- identify the basic requirements for effective communication
- define health communication, health communication and teaching plan
- briefly explain the meaning of the following variables in the health communication process: empathy, control, trust, self-disclosure and confirmation
- identify the core competencies in health education programming
- describe the first step in the planning and evaluation of a health education programme as set out by Ewles and Simnett
- outline the seven steps in the planning and evaluation of a health education programme
- compile a teaching plan for an educational session or intervention.

6.1 INTRODUCTION

Effective communication is a vital requirement for successful coexistence. Not only is this relevant to communication in general, but it also has specific relevance to communication in the health-related environment. All people are born with the gift to communicate, but how effectively this gift is used, depends on many factors. Members of the health team not only have to communicate effectively with patients and the general public, but also need to be able to communicate effectively with other members of the multidisciplinary health team.

All health professionals should acquaint themselves with the nature of the communication process, and should pay attention to aspects such as different communication approaches, basic communication skills, as well as the many factors that could influence effective communication. These aspects form the basis of successful interpersonal relationships, and could affect all situations where there is contact between members of the health team and the community.

6.1.1 The communication process

Communication can be described as the exchange of meaning between two people who strive to reach mutual understanding. Meaning refers not only to factual information included in a particular message, but also to the thoughts, perceptions, ideas and feelings of the various participants in the communication process. Because meaning cannot be transformed from one mind to another, messages must be encoded or given a material form. Encoding can be verbal (spoken or written words) and/or non-verbal (gestures, facial expressions, body language). The transmitted message is then decoded and interpreted by the receiver to give it meaning.

6.1.2 Various means of communication

Messages can be transmitted in more than one way, and the process often occurs in more than one way simultaneously. Communication may be verbal, non-verbal or written communication, and can take place in a formal or informal manner. In addition, even though communication is usually a conscious process, it can, at times, occur unconsciously, where a message is conveyed by means of symbols such as mannerisms, dress or make-up, without the knowledge or conscious effort of the communicator.

Communication can occur in a linear fashion where the communicator, or sender, sends a message to the receiver, or recipient, without allowing for a response or feedback from the recipient who therefore can't express his or her interpretation of the message. This is the style which unfortunately is often used by people in positions of authority, and which definitely does not allow for the free exchange of ideas between all parties concerned. Communication can also occur in a more open and sharing fashion. With such an approach, communication is represented as an interactive or two-way process, characterised by a dynamic process of sharing and feedback.

6.1.3 Communication skills

In addition to the development of skills relevant to verbal, non-verbal or written communication, effective communication also requires the development of other skills, such as understanding, persuasion, motivation, facilitation, reinforcement, reflection, self-disclosure, and most important of all, listening. It is essential that health care professionals make a conscious effort to improve their basic communication skills. There are various opportunities and courses for doing so, both informally in the community, as well as formally, as part of various health-related courses.

6.1.4 Barriers to effective communication

There are many barriers to effective communication. The most common of these include factors relating to individual prejudices, ignorance, language differences, status factors and cultural differences. If, however, we are sincere and honest in our dealings with others, most of these barriers will cease to exist.

It is not intended, nor is it possible, to discuss all the complexities of communication in this chapter. What is intended, however, is to draw the attention to some of the basic requirements for effective communication, and to stimulate the desire to learn more about this very important topic, particularly as it relates to communication in the health-related environment.

6.2 HEALTH COMMUNICATION

Health communication can be defined as the dissemination and interpretation of health-related messages. In this definition the disseminator may be an individual, a group, a mass medium or an organisation, and the interpreter may be a group, an individual, a mass public or an organisation. Health communication, according to Rensburg (1996:211), is a subset of communication which is concerned with how people in a society seek to deal with health-related issues, and to deal with health. The focus in health communication is on health-related transactions, in particular, and on the factors that influence these oral or written, verbal or nonverbal, formal (impersonal) or informal (personal) and relationship-oriented or issue-oriented transactions. Of particular interest in health communication are the transactions that occur between health professionals and clients or patients, and those between health professionals themselves (Rensburg 1996:211-212).

6.2.1 Variables in health communication

Numerous variables are included in the health communication process. These variables affect the health transactions that occur in various health care relationships, and are therefore important to an understanding of the overall health communication process.

For the purpose of this chapter, those variables which are regarded by Rensburg (1996:212-217) as being central to effective health communication, will be explained. These variables are empathy, control, trust, self-disclosure and confirmation.

(a) Empathy

Empathy is regarded as the most essential and at the same time the most complex variable used to explain health communication. Empathy plays an important role in effective interpersonal communication and is believed to affect communication outcomes in all types of relationships. Rensburg (1996:212-213) refers to the definition developed by Carl Rogers which stated that empathy involves a process of "entering the private perceptual world of the other and becoming thoroughly at home in it." Empathy is the sharing of another's feelings, from the other person's point of view.

Empathy is often used interchangeably with sympathy. Empathy is *not* the same as sympathy, because the meanings of these two concepts are very different. Sympathy is the expression of one person's own feeling about another person's predicament. In empathy, the focus is on the client or patient who experiences a problem, whereas with sympathy, the focus shifts away from the client or patient to the health professional. Empathy is important for clients, because ill health is frightening and confusing, and being understood by health professionals helps clients or patients to cope with their emotions. For health professionals, empathy is essential to understand the clients and their problems, as well as to understand other health professionals.

(b) Control

Control is a subtle but powerful factor in health communication, because control forms an integral part of every communication event, and is an intrinsic component of human interaction in general. Whenever a person is influenced by or influences another person or event, aspects of control are present. Control is important to clients or patients, because they are experiencing the loss of it. Loss of control is a problem for the client or patient, because illnesses such as cancer or AIDS, introduce uncertainty into their lives, and with uncertainty comes the loss of control. In turn, loss of control leads to feelings of incompetence, fear, anger or helplessness.

Control is important to health professionals because it is through the negotiation of control that they are able to effectively work with clients or patients and with other members of the multidisciplinary health team. Health professionals therefore need to be sensitive to the effect that loss of control has on clients or patients in the health care setting. Members of the multidisciplinary health team need to restore the client's or patient's sense of control, and not only address the causes of feelings of loss of control.

Being aware of the need for control by clients and health professionals, coupled with flexibility and a willingness to adapt one's own needs for control to the needs of others, will result in better interpersonal communication and more productive relationships between health professional and client (or patient), and between one health professional and another (Rensburg 1996:214).

(c) Trust

Trust is another variable in the health communication process, and involves accepting others without judging or evaluating them. Trust plays an essential part in establishing effective counselling relationships, because it gives relationships a unique, special, positive quality and creates feelings that events are predictable and that individuals are basically sincere, accepting and competent.

In health care, trust is of particular importance to clients or patients, because they frequently feel extremely vulnerable, helpless and in need of support. Clients will feel that they can depend on health professionals to behave in predictable ways and that they can rely on the knowledge and integrity of the members of the multidisciplinary health team. When trust is present in a relationship, a supportive climate is created which reduces defensive communication. Trust helps people to experience a sense of security, a feeling that others care about them. By attending to client or patient's needs and communicating in ways that will create positive reactions, health professionals, as members of the multidisciplinary health team, can foster trust and credibility (Rensburg 1996:214-215).

(d) Self-disclosure

Self-disclosure is the fourth variable in the health communication process and of critical importance in facilitating open communication, which is essential in the development of healthy interpersonal relationships. Self-disclosure may be defined as a process whereby a person communicates personal information, feelings and thoughts, both verbally and nonverbally, to other people.

By becoming more sensitive to the variable of self-disclosure, health professionals and clients can exchange some of their feelings and true concerns. This exchange of feelings and concerns may well result in increased co-operation and understanding among all stakeholders in the health care setting (Rensburg 1996:216).

(e) Confirmation

Confirmation overlaps in some ways with the variables empathy, control, trust and self-disclosure. Rensburg (1996:216) argues that confirmation involves the elements of showing empathy, sharing control, exhibiting trust and disclosing personal feelings and thoughts to others. Rensburg (1996:216) quotes further a suitable description of confirmation made by Northouse and Northouse (1985), namely that confirmation can be described

> "as a means of communicating that focuses on the ways individuals experience the world and ascribe meaning to events. It occurs when individuals respond to others in ways that indicate to others that they are acknowledged and understood."

When health professionals communicate in confirming ways, they provide recognition of clients or patients as unique individuals with real problems. Clients or patients often feel like inanimate objects rather than human beings. One of the reasons for this feeling may be that health professionals themselves receive so little confirmation from clients, patients and other health professionals. Confirmation is not only essential for clients or patients, but is also important for all the members of the multidisciplinary health team.

By communicating in confirming ways, health professionals help clients, patients and other health professionals to cope with feelings of rejection, depersonalisation and even alienation. As Rensburg (1996:217) argues, confirming responses convey to others direct acknowledgement, supportiveness, clarification and expression of positive feelings, and agreement about content of communication messages.

6.3 HEALTH EDUCATION AND HEALTH PROMOTION

During their study on health promotion, Gott and O'Brien (1990:142) encountered the frequent practice of referring to and interpreting health promotion and health education as one and the same. They argued that it is assumed that:

- health education and health promotion are one and the same
- health promotion is only about getting people to do "healthy things"
- people can and will change their behaviour because a nurse tells them to.

The African National Congress also expressed its concern by stating in the National Health Plan for South Africa (ANC 1994(a):41), that "health promotion is not well understood in South Africa and many people equate health promotion with health education."

The terms "health promotion" and "health education" are not interchangeable. Health promotion covers all aspects of those activities that seek to improve the health status of communities and individuals. It includes both health education and all attempts to produce environmental and legislative change conducive to good health. Hence, health promotion is concerned with making healthier choices easier choices (Webb 1994:16).

Ewles and Simnett (1992) claim that knowledge is a basic human right and if education is required to obtain it, then all means should be taken to bring this about. They go on to say that, without knowledge, people cannot make healthy choices about their own lifestyles or be equipped for social and political lobbying to change things for society generally. Health education has, self-evidently, been concerned with influencing health choices throughout its history, but in fact education for health is an essential prerequisite in all health promotion programmes. Wilson-Barnett and Clark (1993:3) encapsulated the structural analysis of health promotion in a simple formula: "Health promotion = health education × healthy public policy."

The relationship between health education and the process of building healthy public policy is viewed by Tone *et al.* (1990:4) as symbiotic. They argue that health promotion is an amalgam of policy development and health education. Health promotion, therefore, consists of any combination of education and related environmental, economic, legal, fiscal and organisational interventions designed to facilitate the achievement of health.

Because people have the right to be involved in both the planning and implementation of their health care, which includes health education, we need to take a closer look at the meaning of health education.

6.4 WHAT IS HEALTH EDUCATION?

Health education assists people to facilitate changes to more helpful behaviours. This may be achieved through the use of the educational process by a variety of learning experiences.

Catford and Nutbeam (1984:7) made the following statement on their view of health education:

- Health education seeks to improve or protect health through voluntary changes in behaviours as a sequence of learning opportunities
- Health education can include
  - personal education and development
  - mass media information.

Personal education and development concerns improving knowledge about health, promoting self-empowerment and self-esteem, and offering health-risk advice through health professional-client/patient contacts.

Mass media information and education tend to be non-personal and concern raising public awareness, offering health-risk advice and information, and creating a climate of opinion, through news information, distance learning projects and advertising, e.g. through television, radio and newspapers.

With an empowerment approach, as explained in the previous chapter, education becomes a dynamic process involving critical examination of received wisdom and taken-for-granted beliefs and values. In health promotion terms, according to Williams (1995:38), it becomes a means of enabling people to explore health as a social and political issue, and to challenge the way in which health problems are conceptualised in individualistic terms, and the social structural causes ignored or denied.

The interpretation of health education is open to many kinds of criticism. Tone and Tilford (1994:11) developed the following technical definition, a definition that still holds true.

> "Health education is any intentional activity which is designed to achieve health or illness related learning, i.e. some relatively permanent change in an individual's capability or disposition. Effective health education may thus produce changes in knowledge and understanding or ways of thinking; it may influence or clarify values; it may bring about some shift in belief or attitude; it may facilitate the acquisition of skills; it may even effect changes in behaviour or lifestyle."

Health education, in addition, is a process that frees people to voluntarily adopt or alter behaviours that will improve or maintain their health.

Health education can thus be viewed as the process of influencing behaviour and producing changes in knowledge, attitudes and skills required to improve and maintain health, by the use of the education process.

The goal of health education is to make the client (community, group, individual) part of the education process in order that the information provided can be used to enhance its health status. Health education requires an ongoing assessment of the client's attitudes, knowledge and skills, because it occurs over a period of time (Rankin and Stallings 1990:85–6).

6.5 HEALTH EDUCATION PROGRAMMES

For the purpose of this chapter, emphasis will be placed on the one positive health activity, namely health education programmes.

By implementing the Reconstruction and Development Programme (RDP) and the National Health Plan (NHP), the Government of National Unity committed itself to the promotion of health for all the people of South Africa, through

> "prevention and education. Health workers at all levels will promote general health and encourage healthy lifestyles. The government will also seek to establish appropriate mechanisms that will lead to the integration of traditional and other complementary healers into the NHS." (ANC 1994(a):50; ANC 1994(b):20).

To give emphasis to the establishment of "appropriate mechanisms" to promote health, health education programmes will be highlighted in more detail. All community health practitioners will benefit from detailed information on the development of health education programmes. The WHO expressed its concern about the importance of education on health, by ranking "education concerning prevailing health problems and the methods of preventing and controlling them" (WHO 1978:4) as the first element of primary health care.

A programme can be described as a standing arrangement that provides a social service. Health education programmes are planned opportunities for people to learn about health and to undertake voluntary changes in their behaviour with regard to health. Health education programmes may include providing information, exploring attitudes and values, making health decisions and acquiring skills to enable behavioural change to take place. Such programmes involve promoting self-empowerment and self-esteem so that people are enabled to take action about their health (Hayes and Fors 1990:208–11).

Health education in health education programmes can take place on a personal level, such as in the relationship between a community health nurse and client, on a group level, such as in an antenatal exercise class, or by means of reaching large audiences through the mass media, exhibitions and health fairs.

As indicated in Figure 6.1, health education programmes may also be part of personal services, social services and health care. Because of this, the concepts of primary, secondary and tertiary health education should be explained:

- Primary health education is concerned with positively improving the quality of health, as well as the quality of life, and not merely preventing illness. Primary health education is directed towards healthy people and aims to prevent ill health.
- Secondary health education is directed towards people who are ill and is concerned with educating them about their condition and how to deal with it. Restoring good health may involve the client in changing behaviour or in complying with a therapeutic regimen. Secondary health education may involve the client in learning about self-care and self-help.
- Tertiary health education is directed towards clients whose ill health has not been, or could not be, prevented and who cannot be completely cured. Tertiary health education is concerned with educating those clients and their relatives on how to make the most of their remaining potential for healthy living. Rehabilitation programmes on how to avoid unnecessary hardship, restrictions and complications, contain a considerable amount of tertiary health education. It should be mentioned that it is not always easy to see where people fit into primary, secondary or tertiary health education because a person's state of health is open to interpretation.

Having identified that health education, expressed in health education programmes, is a positive health promotion activity, we need to look at the skills and methods used to put it into action.

6.6 CORE COMPETENCIES IN HEALTH EDUCATION PROGRAMMING

Ewles and Simnett (1992:27–9) identified six areas of core competencies in health that can be applied to health education programmes for health promotion.

These competencies are illustrated in Figure 6.1.

FIGURE 6.1: Core competencies in health education programming

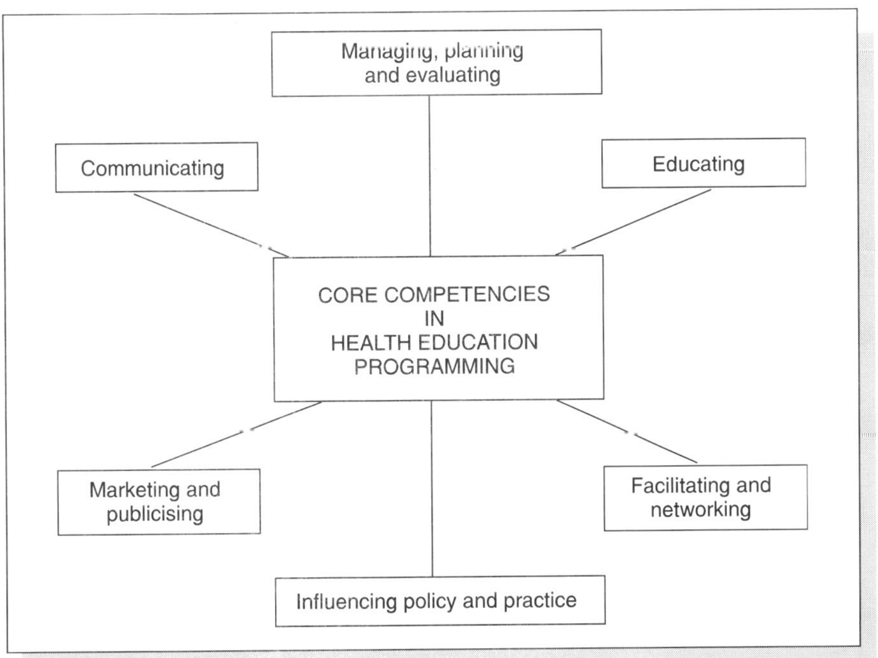

Source: Ewles and Simnett (1992:29)

- *Managing, planning and evaluating.* Effective and efficient health education programmes need systematic planning and managing of resources such as money, manpower, facilities and equipment. All positive health activities need evaluation.
- *Communicating.* Competent communication is essential, because health education means working with people in a one-on-one situation or with groups in various formal and informal ways.

- *Educating*. Teaching about health requires good communication but also additional educational competence, because health educators have to work in different settings such as group discussions, formal lectures or informal groups.
- *Marketing and publicising*. These competencies would, for example, enrol local radio and the local press in giving coverage to health issues which would benefit from wider publicity.
- *Facilitating and networking*. When working with communities, these competencies will help people promote their own health and that of others by sharing skills and information and consequently building up trust and confidence.
- *Influencing policy and practice*. Health educators influence broad plans of action and practices which affect health.

The community health nurse, in the role of health educator, needs a high level of competence in communication and education. She also needs the competencies of facilitating and networking in order to plan and evaluate her health education, market the health education programmes to her clients, facilitate change and be able to refer the client to other helpful sectors in the community's network.

All six of these areas of competence are fundamental to health promotion activities.

6.7 PLANNING AND EVALUATING HEALTH EDUCATION PROGRAMMES

Since health is considered a fundamental human right, it can be argued that communities, groups, families and individuals can do something to improve their own health and that they may want to take responsibility for themselves. Sensitive and well-planned health education programmes can promote people's confidence and self-esteem, empowering them to take more control over their own health.

The planning of a health education programme is a collaborative and systematic process which ends with a plan to attain certain set goals. Adequate planning should assure people that they will have input into organised health education efforts. With systematic planning, limited resources are used most effectively and people are allowed to feel that they are in control.

The planning process, ending with a plan, should give answers to the following three questions:

- What are we trying to achieve?
- What are we going to do?
- How will we know whether we have been successful?

The first question, "What are we trying to achieve?", is concerned with identifying needs and priorities and being clear about specific aims and objectives, while the second question, "What are we going to do?", suggests the following steps:

- selecting the best way of achieving the aims from various possibilities
- identifying the resources that are going to be used
- setting a clear action plan of who does what and when.

The third question, "How will we know whether we have been successful?", highlights the need for evaluation to be included. Evaluation forms an integral part of the overall health education programme.

FIGURE 6.2: A flow diagram for the planning and evaluation of a health education programme

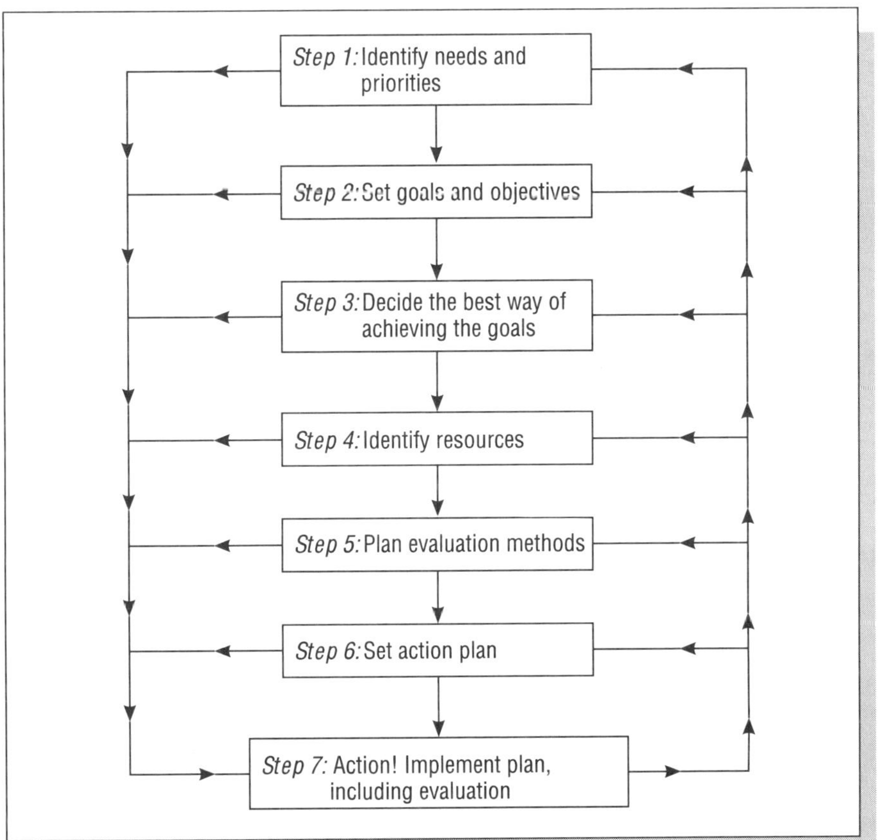

Source: Ewles and Simnett (1992:85)

A seven-step flow diagram (Figure 6.2) provides the answer to these questions with their concerns. Note that the arrows on the diagram lead one's thinking in a circle. This makes it possible to rethink and change original ideas as the plan and evaluation are carried out. The main direction of the arrows is anticlockwise, indicating that in reality planning is not a tidy process. In fact, one could continually review, change and improve the plan, using the diagram to keep one on course.

Step 1: identifying needs and priorities

Identifying people's needs and prioritising them is a difficult process. An even more complex process is identifying the people who are intended to benefit from health education programmes as a health promotion activity. Some people are referred to as "users" of community health services, while other people are called "receivers", because they "receive" help rather than "use" it.

It is, however, important to keep in mind that it is just as essential to identify potential users as it is to identify current users. Therefore, it might be necessary to take positive action so that some people do not get more out of existing community health services than others.

A closer look at the bottomless pit of needs reveals that needs can be classified in four categories:

- *Felt need*. A need in which people identify what they want.
- *Expressed need*. What people say they need. This is felt need which has been turned into an expressed request or demand.
- *Normative need*. A need defined by a professional or expert, based on value judgement and standards according to professional experts.
- *Comparative need*. A comparative need for health education programmes is defined by comparing similar groups of clients, some of whom are part of health education programmes and others who are not.

Needs assessment includes consideration of the needs and interests of the community as a whole, the people being served and the community health service. Needs assessment also includes learning about the client's culture, health beliefs, health behaviour, experience, skills and attitudes (McAllister and Farquhar 1992:1447–9).

In addition to the basic definitions of health, wellness and need, experts in the field of wellness present various approaches to health and wellness. These approaches are referred to as conceptual models, and provide a viewpoint or structure from which to organise global ideas about groups, individuals and situations in a meaningful way and to guide the thinking, interpretations and observations of people on health.

In community health nursing, the PRECEDE model and the health belief model are especially applicable to the task of health education as part of the educating role of the community health nurse.

(a) The PRECEDE model

This health education planning model is depicted in Figure 6.3. PRECEDE stands for predisposing, reinforcing and enabling causes in educational diagnosis and evaluation. The model is based on the theory that because health and health behaviour are determined by several factors, health education efforts to change behaviour must be multidimensional. It shows that certain environmental factors motivate people to exhibit certain health behaviours. The model uses a problem-solving approach and focuses on helping groups to change behaviours.

FIGURE 6.3: The PRECEDE model

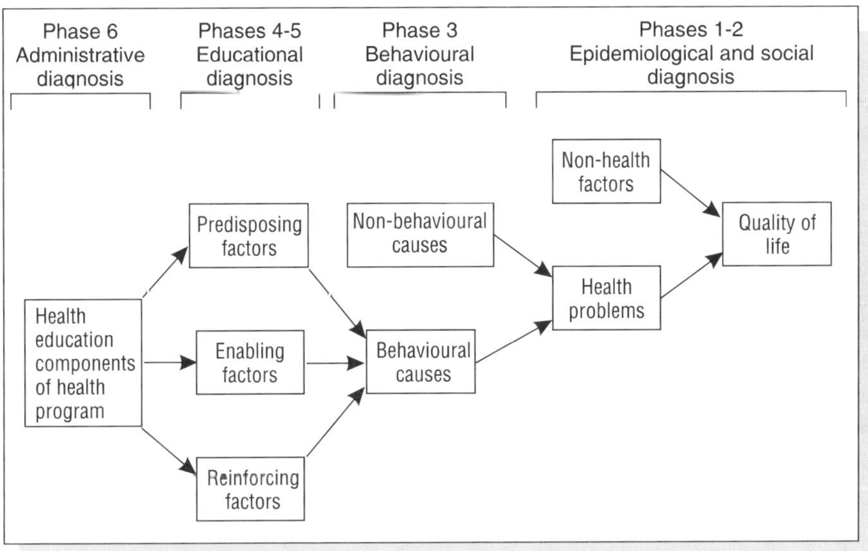

Source: Redman (1993:19)

The PRECEDE model is easy to use; it starts with a process of considering desired outcomes and works back to original causes. The model is applied in the following phases:

Phase 1: Consider the quality of life of the group or individual involved.

Phase 2: Identify specific health problems contributing to the social problem identified in phase 1.

Phase 3: Identify specific health-related behaviours associated with the identified health problems.

Phase 4: Categorise the factors that have a direct impact on the behaviour selected:

- *Predisposing factors*: factors internal to the client, such as values,

beliefs, attitudes and perceptions which facilitate or hinder motivation
- *Enabling factors*: barriers created by forces external to the client
- *Reinforcing factors*: forces external to the client and related to the feedback the client receives from others, be it positive or negative.

Phase 5: Decide which factors will be the focus of intervention.
Phase 6: Select interventions and assess administrative problems and resources.
Phase 7: Evaluate.

(b) Health belief model

The health belief model attempts to explain why and under what conditions people take action to detect, prevent or comply with treatment. The model was developed to provide a framework to explain why some people take specific action to avoid illness, while others fail to protect themselves.

In community health nursing, the health belief model is useful in looking at health-protecting or disease-preventing behaviour. The model asserts that the motivation for people to take action to promote health or to prevent disease is based on how strongly they believe that:
- they are susceptible to the disease in question
- the disease would have serious effects on their lives if they should contract it
- the suggested health intervention is of value
- the effectiveness of the treatment is worth the cost and barriers they must confront.

The health belief model is useful in organising information about clients' views of their state of health and what factors would influence them to change their behaviour. The model is divided into three major components: individual perceptions, modifying factors and variables affecting the likelihood of initiating actions (Figure 6.4).

Health education can be developed on the basis of data gathered from the model for looking at client status. For example, if a community refuses to make use of the family planning service, the health belief model could be used to determine the clients' perception of the risk of taking contraceptives, their knowledge of family planning (services) and their views of what might be the advantages and disadvantages of family planning. Group or individual instruction could be instituted that would clarify any misconceptions and provide essential health information found lacking in the assessment of perceptions and benefits of actions (Stanhope and Lancaster 1992:187).

FIGURE 6.4: The health belief model

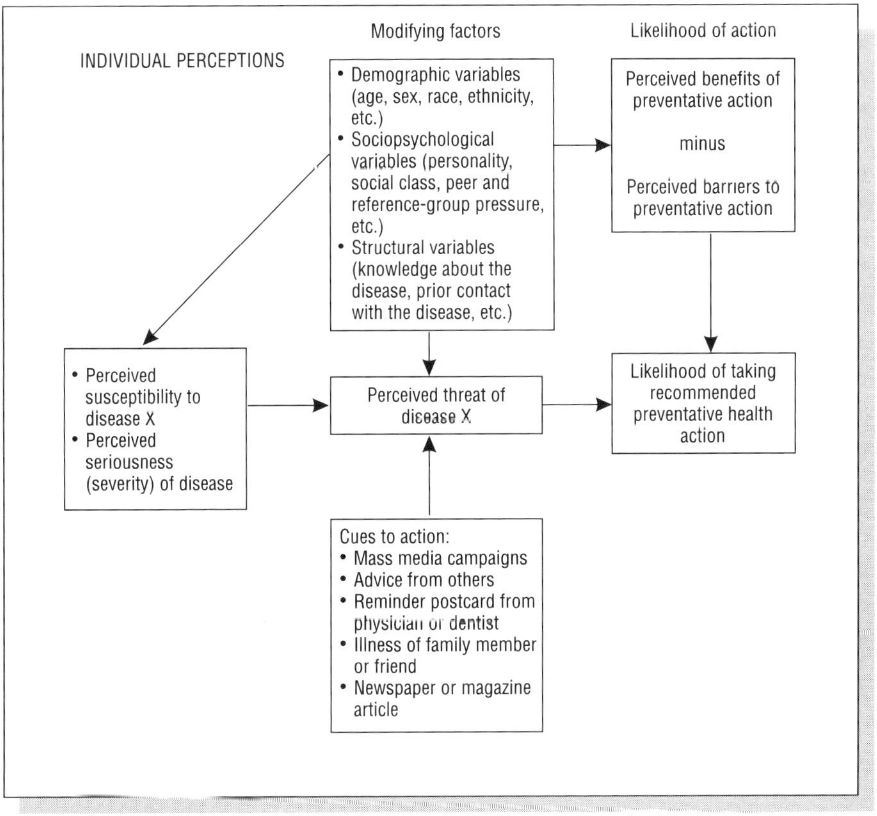

Source: Cookfair (1991:72)

Step 2: setting goals and objectives

Having assessed the client's needs for the health education programme, the overall goals and objectives of the programme are established.

Goals are broad statements of what is going to be achieved by the health education programme, while objectives are more specific. Objectives are written statements of expected outcome, or change in behaviour to be achieved within a specified period. Objectives have additional characteristics. They should be:

- attainable and realistic
- challenging
- as measurable as possible
- consistent with the goals of the comprehensive community health service rendered locally.

For programme objectives to be useful, they should meet several criteria, namely (Clark 1992:441):

- measurability
- reasonability or practicality
- time specificity
- being within group competencies
- congruence with community morals
- legality
- acceptability to implementers
- fitting budgetary limitations
- carrying minimal side-effects.

Step 3: determining the best way of achieving the goals

There is a range of possible ways of accomplishing the formulated goals and objectives. But there is no one best way to go about a health education programme or health promotion as a whole.

Some factors to consider include:

- Which methods are most appropriate and effective in achieving the goals and objectives?
- Which methods are most acceptable to the people involved?
- Which methods are most acceptable to the client?
- Which methods will be the easiest, cheapest and most comfortable to use?

A number of goals, grouped into categories with effective and appropriate methods for achieving them, are identified in Table 6.1.

Step 4: identifying resources

Once goals and objectives have been established, the planning process can proceed to identify resources needed to implement the health education programme.

In an attempt to clarify what resources are needed, what resources are going to be used and what additional resources are to be acquired, the following kinds of resources given by Ewles and Simnett (1992:92) may serve as a guideline:

- *Professional health practitioners:* their skills, knowledge, experience, energy, enthusiasm and time are vital resources.
- *The client* (community, group, family, aggregate or individual): clients may have knowledge, skills, energy, enthusiasm and time which can be used to build upon. In this way clients can help each other to learn and change.
- *People who can help*: may include colleagues, other health workers, people with relevant expertise and lay people who have something to offer.
- *People who influence the client*: may include other clients, relatives, friends, care groups, self-help groups and volunteers.

TABLE 6.1: Goals and methods in health education programmes

Goal	Appropriate method
Health awareness goal Raising awareness or consciousness of health issues	Talks Group discussion Campaigns Exhibitions Mass media
Self-empowering Improving self-esteem, decision-making, self-awareness	Group work Values clarification Practising decision-making Role-play, simulation Counselling
Changing attitudes and behaviour Changing lifestyles	Group discussion Self-help groups One-on-one instruction Advice Mass media
Improving knowledge Providing information	Group teaching One-on-one teaching Mass media Written material Displays and exhibitions
Societal or environmental change Changing the social or physical environment	Positive action for underserved groups Community development Advocacy schemes Enforcement of laws and regulations

Source: Ewles and Simnett (1992:91)

- *Existing services and facilities*: what are the existing services and facilities and how are these utilised?
- *Existing policies and plans*: what policies and plans on health promotion issues exist and can be used to back up the planned health education programme?
- *Material resources*: these include venues, space, seats, audiovisual equipment, printed material, posters and display material.

Step 5: planning evaluation methods

Once a detailed plan for the health education programme has been constructed, and specific activities delineated, the plan itself should be evaluated.

Evaluation simply means making a judgement on the value of something.

In this case, it means looking critically at the health education programme. Programmes are evaluated to decide what was good about them, what was bad and how they could be improved. Evaluation is thus the process of assessing what was achieved and how it was achieved.

The judgement of the value of the programme can be about the outcome; what was achieved, and about the process; indicating how it was achieved. Evaluation should be non-threatening, because it implies a willingness to change, a desire to improve. If evaluation is used positively, it can be viewed as an opportunity to improve a programme as it develops and as an opportunity to measure success, and not failure.

Evaluation requires sound planning skills and a commitment not to manipulate the outcome.

(a) Assessing the outcome

Outcome evaluation, or judging what has been achieved, focuses on the extent to which the goals and objectives of the health education programme have been met, irrespective of how well organised or how efficient the programme was. As Clark (1992:444) justly remarks, outcome evaluation documents the effects of the programme and justifies decisions to continue, to modify or to eliminate it.

The type of changes which may be reflected in the objectives and methods that might be used to assess or measure those changes are indicated in Table 6.2.

(b) Assessing the process

Process evaluation is concerned with the smoothness of operation of the programme, which means assessing the degree to which objectives are met or planned and activities are conducted.

Process evaluation examines programme performance by looking at what went on during the process of implementation, and making judgements about it. Programme performance can be assessed by:

- *Measuring the input or effort* to make judgements as to whether the outcome was worthwhile. Everything that went into the health education programme in terms of time, materials and money, has to be recorded.
- *Self-evaluation.* Ask yourself what you did well, or what you would like to change. Emphasise the positive and look for constructive ways for aspects to be improved.
- *Feedback from other people.* Asking questions and getting feedback from clients and peers are essential skills for every health educator. Obtaining feedback from the client should be part of assessing the process of every

nursing intervention, while getting feedback from a colleague on work performance is a valuable form of peer evaluation.

TABLE 6.2: Changes and methods to assess or measure them

Types of change	Methods to assess or measure the change
Change in health awareness	Measuring the interest shown by consumers Monitoring changes in demand for health-related services Analysis of media coverage Interviews, questionnaires, observation with groups or individuals, discussion
Behavioural change	Observing what clients do Recording behaviour, e.g. • regular recording of numbers attending clinic • periodic inventory by follow-up questionnaires or interviews
Change in knowledge or attitude	Observing change in what clients do and say Interviews and discussions: question-and-answer between health educator and clients Observation of how clients apply knowledge to real-life situations Discussion on how clients solve problems
Change in health status	Keeping records of health indicators – growth charts, mass, blood pressure Health surveys to identify larger-scale changes in health behaviour Analysis of trends in health statistics such as morbidity or infant mortality rates

Source: Ewles and Simnett (1992:96)

Step 6: setting an action plan

By setting an action plan, one is at the stage where one knows:

- what is going to be achieved
- what is the best way to go about it
- how to evaluate process and outcome
- what resources are needed.

Setting an action plan means writing a detailed statement of who will do what, by when, how, where and with what resources.

It is helpful to break down the plan into manageable elements or key events. When drawing up a schedule that shows the key events, deadlines should be specified that must be met by the people involved.

Step 7: action

Step 7 indicates the stage at which the health education programme is actually put into operation, evaluating the process as it goes along.

Ewles and Simnett (1992:99) give an outline to put ideas into action when planning a health education programme (Table 6.3).

TABLE 6.3: Ideas into action: planning a health education programme

Work alone or in a small group.

Think of an area of health education within your scope of practice as a health practitioner where there is a need for health promotion. It could be an established area of work such as a community health clinic, a school health service or occupational health services.

Work through the following steps of the planning cycle. Start by writing each of the following headings at the top of a separate sheet of paper, and then work through them:

1. *Aim and objectives*. Identify the broad aim(s), and be more specific in identifying and formulating the objectives. Ask yourself, "What am I trying to achieve?"
2. *The best way of achieving aims and objectives*. Think of all the ways in which aims and objectives can be achieved and identify the best way.
3. *Resources*. Identify resources that are already available and others that are needed.
4. *Evaluation*. Identify how both the process and outcome of the programme will be evaluated. Ask yourself, "How will I know if I am successful?"
5. *Action plan*. Identify who will do what, by when, how, where and with what resources.

The findings of the outcome and process evaluation are used to make decisions about the health education programme. The decisions that can be made, based on evaluating findings, are: to continue, to modify or to discontinue the programme.

When the decision is made that the health education programme should continue, the action plan is put into practice by a group of people who serve as a communication network.

6.8 TEACHING PLAN

Community health practitioners, particularly the community health nurse, work with groups. In their daily practice, they plan and implement health-focused interventions with clients, with colleagues and other members of the interdisciplinary health team. Community health nurses often participate in groups and are called upon to initiate and direct group problem-solving activities. They must be conversant with the processes that govern the operation of groups. Community health nurses need group-process skills to empower people (the community and individuals) to increase control over, and improve, their health.

Health education is an activity that cannot be indulged in without prior planning, and so is teaching. Teaching is an intentional enterprise with the aim of facilitating other people's learning. Professional teaching, as explained by Quinn (1995:113), is characterised by an acceptance of responsibility for facilitating other people's learning through planned and purposeful educational interventions. These educational interventions or teaching sessions may form part of a health education programme. During an educational intervention between *teacher* and *learner*, the use of a teaching plan can help to minimise the chances of omitting some vital part of the health education session, and ensure that all the necessary factors have been considered.

A teacher needs to spend time and energy on the preparation of an educational intervention, so as to be able to give a stimulating performance. The teacher must know how to present materials so that the learners will perceive the relationship of the educational material to the objectives and, at the same time, keep interest at a level that will help the learner to pursue the objectives. The teacher must guide and assist the learner until the objectives are reached. The teacher plans ways to attain the objectives formulated for the educational intervention.

Only through planning can the teacher be certain that the significant ideas, knowledge and details are included to help the learner attain the objectives. The need to plan for teaching is evident (Guinée 1966:91-92).

According to Redman (1993:196), teaching plans can be written in many formats, but the major criterion in judging the format is whether it facilitates the relationship between its parts.

The format for a teaching plan (Figure 6.5) outlines the parts of a teaching plan. Teaching plans specify guidelines, but must be adapted to the individual client, patients, group, aggregates or the community itself.

Standardised teaching plans are excellent if used properly. They are developed to be used as guides to client, patient or group teaching. Since clients and patients are people with different health needs and abilities, these teaching plans must be adapted. Standard teaching plans serve to save interventions to meet individual client, patient or group needs (Anderson 1990:176).

As developed by Quinn (1995:124), Figure 6.5 gives a framework for a teaching plan which will suit any type of teaching situation. It fits neatly on to

FIGURE 6.5: Format for a teaching plan

Title (topic) ....

Date ....

Teaching method:
(e.g lecture, demonstration, group discussion)

....

Time ....

Venue ....

GROUP DETAILS	
(a) Number of learners	
(b) Type of educational session/intervention	
(c) Subject	
(d) Educational level	
(e) Previous experience	
ROOM ARRANGEMENTS	TEACHING AIDS
Chairs, adequate light and ventilation, technical media in working order	Transparencies, chalk-board, hand notes, pamphlets
EVALUATION FORMAT	
(a) During session	(b) End of session
AIMS AND OBJECTIVES	
OUTLINE OF SESSION /LESSON	

TIME	SEQUENCE	ACTIVITY	
		TEACHER	LEARNERS

Source: Adapted from Quinn (1995:124, in Unisa NUE100-6/105/98:95)

TABLE 6.4 : Outline of an educational session or intervention

Time	Sequence	Teacher activity	Learner activity
3 minutes	**Introduction to the topic** Asking questions Refer to objects (where applicable)	Tell something to rouse interest Link, e.g a story to the topic Ask questions to activate thinking Announce topic Explain object (where applicable)	Listen Active thinking and answering questions Listen Take notes (if applicable)
2 minutes	**Pre-knowledge testing** Asking questions Use of media	Use media and questions to recall previous knowledge	Active thinking and recall of knowledge Answering Active involvement
27 minutes	**New contents** Explanation by use of media: – write on chalkboard – transparencies, videos, pictures, etc. Asking questions Show real object (where applicable)	List and define terms Exposition of new contents by interpretive explanation Use media to reinforce contents Questions to recall previous knowledge Questions to stimulate thinking Use of media – real object Questions to activate thinking Using examples Questions to test insight and understanding	Active thinking Answering Listen and observe Taking notes (where applicable) Active thinking
3 minutes	**Summary** Using media – or headings on chalkboard	Repetition of main points to reinforce	Listening
4 minutes	**Evaluation** Prepare questions you want to ask with the answers	Ask questions to test understanding and insight	Active thinking Answering

Source: Unisa (NUE100-6/105/98:99-105)

an A4 sheet and contains spaces for all the necessary details on one side, with room for the actual sequence of delivery on the reverse. Most of the framework is self-explanatory, but the following should be noted.

The column headed sequence of the lesson is for the main headings of the teaching session or educational intervention. The activity column is an useful indicator of the amount of activity or interaction during the educational intervention or teaching session, and should also include any use of learning resources as well as teacher talk. The time column is included to be an approximate guide, and the plan must be flexible to allow for unplanned events.

6.9 SUMMARY

Health promotion is viewed as an umbrella term, encompassing health education programmes as a positive activity for better health. Health education is referred to as a central tool in health promotion, a tool to empower people to make healthier choices more easily and to increase control over the determinants of health, and thereby improve health.

Health education ceases to be an instrument of social control and becomes a means of social change. This can also be applied to health education. It is the nature of empowerment education, a concept which has now been taken up in health education and health promotion (Williams 1995:38).

In this chapter the PRECEDE model and the Health Belief model are explained because both models are applicable to health education as part of the educating role of health professionals, and in particular that of the community nurse.

To plan effective health educational session or interventions with clients, groups, aggregates and the community itself, the use of a teaching plan can help to ensure that the necessary factors have been considered, and to minimise the chances of omitting some vital part of the health education session or intervention. A format for a teaching plan is included and the outline of an educational session or intervention is given, which may serve as a framework for an education session.

Bibliography

African National Congress. 1994(a). *A national health plan for South Africa.* Maseru: Bähr Mapping and Printing.

African National Congress. 1994(b). *The reconstruction and development programme.* Johannesburg: Umanyano.

Anderson, C. 1990. *Patient teaching and communicating in a informal age.* New York: Demar Publishers.

Catford, J. and Nutbeam, D. 1984. Towards a definition of health education and health promotion. *Health education journal.* Vol. 43, Nos. 2&3:7.

Clark, M.J. 1992. *Nursing in the community.* Norwalk: Appleton and Lange.

Cookfair, J.M. 1991. *Nursing process and the practical in the community.* St Louis: Mosby.

Ewles, L. and Simnett, I. 1992. *Promoting health: a practical guide.* 2nd ed. London: Scutari Press.

Gott, M. and O'Brien, M. 1990. The role of the nurse in health promotion. *Health promotion international.* Vol. 5, No. 2:137–43.

Guinée, K. 1966. *The aims and methods of nursing education.* New York: Macmillan.

Hayes, D.M. and Fors, S.W. 1990. Self-esteem and health instruction: challenges for curriculum development. *Journal of school health.* May, Vol. 60, No. 5:208–9.

McAllister, G. and Farquhar, M. 1992. Health beliefs: a cultural division? *Journal of advanced nursing.* Vol. 17: 1447–54.

Northouse, P.G. and Northouse, L.L. 1985. *Health communication. A handbook for health professionals.* Englewood Clifs, NJ: Prentice-Hall.

Quinn, F.M. 1995. *The principles and practice of nurse education.* 3rd ed. London: Chapman and Hall.

Rankin, S.H. and Stallings, K.D. 1990. *Patient education: issues, principles, practices.* 2nd ed. Philadelphia: Lippencott.

Redman, B.K. 1993. *The process of patient teaching.* St Louis: Mosby.

Rensburg, R.S. (Ed.) 1996. *Introduction to communication: communication planning and management.* Course book 4. Kenwyn: Juta.

Stanhope, M.E. and Lancaster, J. 1992. *Community health nursing: process and practice for promoting health.* St Louis: Mosby.

Tone, K., Tilford, S. and Robinson, Y. 1990, 1994. *Health education: effectiveness and efficiency.* London: Chapman and Hall.

University of South Africa. Department of Advanced Nursing Sciences. 1998. *Nursing Education 1: tutorial letter.* 105/1998 for NUE 100–6. Pretoria.

Webb, P. 1994. *Health promotion and patient education.* London: Chapman and Hall.

Williams, J. 1995. Education for empowerment: implications for professional development and training in health promotion. *Health education journal.* Vol. 54:37–47.

Wilson-Barnett, J. and Clark, J.M. 1993. *Research in health promotion and nursing.* London: Macmillan.

World Health Organisation. 1978. *Primary health care. Report of the international conference on primary health care.* Alma-Ata, USSR. 6–12 September 1978. Geneva.

World Health Organisation. 1984. *Health promotion: a discussion document on the concepts and principles*. Copenhagen: WHO Regional Office for Europe.

World Health Organisation. 1986. *Ottawa charter for health promotion: an international conference on health promotion*. November 17–21. Copenhagen: WHO Regional Office for Europe.

World Health Organisation. 1987. *Health promotion: concepts and principles in action, a policy framework*. Copenhagen: WHO Regional Office for Europe.

World Health Organisation. 1988. *From Alma-Ata to the year 2000: reflections at the midpoint*. Geneva: WHO.

Yeo, M. 1993. Towards an ethic of empowerment for health promotion. *Health promotion international*. Vol. 8, No. 3:225–35.

7

Strategies for the transformation of the health system in South Africa

KATHLEEN DENNILL

"The time for the healing of the wounds is come. The moment to bridge the chasms that divide us has come. The time to build is upon us." (Nelson Mandela: 1994.05.10)

CHAPTER OBJECTIVES

After reading this chapter, the student should be able to:

- discuss the health vision and the health system of South Africa
- explain the strategic planning process and how it can be applied to the implementation of primary health care programmes
- discuss legislation which both impacts on and enables the implementation of primary health care
- discuss various health policies and, through this process, determine how the policies are influencing the delivery and the success of primary health care programmes in South Africa
- understand what is meant by the district health system, and discuss the process being followed to implement such a system in South Africa.

7.1 INTRODUCTION

Progress towards the attainment of "health for all" requires the appropriate organisation and management of health systems. For these processes to be successful, they must be dynamic and goal-driven, based on both the ongoing assessment of the environment and a "health" vision for the future. The strategies of action selected to reach the determined health-related goals, must take into consideration both the strengths and weaknesses of the total environment and should be developed to support the effective and efficient delivery of health services. The chosen strategies are the basis for major policy and practice decisions and are determined by the government in power. The successful implementation of these strategies will, however, depend on input from, and ownership by, all the relevant role-players in the extended multidisciplinary health team.

On 27 April 1995, the African National Congress came into power, with a new health vision for South Africa - a unified health system based on comprehensive primary health care and where "... resources are rationally and effectively used, to make basic health care available to all South Africans, giving priority to the most vulnerable groups" (ANC 1994(a):20).

In April 1997 the White Paper for the Transformation of the Health System in South Africa was published by the Ministry of Health. It contains the policy objectives and principles upon which the Unified Health System of South Africa is based. It also contains implementation strategies to meet the basic needs of the South African people, within the constraints determined by the limited available resources, and within both the public and private health sectors.

In this chapter health planning and health management for primary health care will be discussed, subject to the health policy decisions as well as the strategies determined to implement the new health system in South Africa. The expectations of the recipients of health care and the realities of the process of implementing the Unified Health System of South Africa, will also be discussed.

7.2 THE MISSION AND OBJECTIVES OF THE SOUTH AFRICAN NATIONAL HEALTH SYSTEM

In the introduction to the White Paper, the Minister of Health, Dr Nkosazana Zuma (Republic of South Africa 1997:5) refers to the task of "developing a unified health system capable of delivering quality health care to all our citizens efficiently and in a caring environment". The system will be based on comprehensive primary health care and will include a national socio-economic development programme, the Reconstruction and Development Programme.

MISSION STATEMENT OF THE DEPARTMENT OF HEALTH

To provide leadership and guidance to the National Health System in its efforts to promote and monitor the health of all people in South Africa, and to provide caring and effective services through the primary health care approach.

Source: Republic of South Africa (1997:13)

The objectives of restructuring the Health System (Republic of South Africa 1997:14-16), as set out in the White Paper, are to:

(a) Unify fragmented health services at all levels into a comprehensive and integrated National Health Service.
(b) Promote equity, accessibility and utilisation of health services.
(c) Extend the availability and ensure the appropriateness of health services.
(d) Develop health promotion activities.
(e) Develop the human resources available to the health sector.
(f) Foster community participation across the health sector.
(g) Improve health sector planning and monitoring of health status and services.

To attain these objectives, implementation strategies have been identified, policies developed and a process of implementation agreed upon. However, the process is dynamic and will need to adapt as the environment or the needs of the people change.

7.3 THE STRATEGIC PLANNING PROCESS

South Africa's social and political transition, and the process of democratising both the State and society, have provided opportunities for change in the health sector which have rarely been available to any country. Active participation of all sectors of South African society, including the community, has been sought in the development of strategies to improve the health of the people.

To this end health services are in the process of being restructured with the aim of attaining equity in accessibility to health services for all the people of the country. The emphasis of the new health policy is to move away from a curative and urban-centred health system to one based on a comprehensive primary health care approach. The fragmentation of services inherited from the previous government, and a lack of appropriately trained managers, have been two important factors that have inhibited the progress of the transformation.

Strategic planning is a management skill that health care providers need to acquire. Whether at national, provincial or district level, the health care provider who is responsible for implementing health policy will be required to develop strategies pertinent to the specific needs of that region, area or community.

The art of strategic planning is well defined by Evashwick and Evashwick (Spiegal and Hyman 1991:4), when they say that:

> "Strategic planning is the process of assessing a changing environment to create a vision of the future; determining how the organisation fits into the anticipated environment based on its institutional mission, strengths and weaknesses; and then setting in motion a plan of action to position the organisation accordingly."

Another simple way of explaining the essence of strategic planning is to ask the following questions about the organisation or work situation: Where are we now? Where do we wish to go? How will we get there? It is a problem-solving process which requires both judgement and technique.

In the health planning process, there are two terms or concepts used extensively, namely strategic planning and comprehensive health planning. There is little difference in the meaning of these terms, except perhaps in the philosophy that underlies the two concepts:

- *Strategic planning* focuses on the survival of the organisation, since it endeavours to provide services to the health and welfare of the public.
- *Comprehensive health planning* is concerned with the health, medical and welfare needs of the people, regardless of the profit or loss aspect.

The actual process of strategic health planning varies from situation to situation, but according to Simyar *et al.* (Spiegal and Hyman 1991:6) there are eight steps in the strategic health planning process that can be applied to most situations. These steps are to:

- identify the organisation's current position, including its current mission statement, and long-term objectives and policies
- analyse the environment, both internal and external, in which the organisation functions
- conduct an organisational audit to identify both the current position and the desired position of the organisation
- identify alternative strategies based on the relevant data to reach the identified desired position
- select the best alternative/s, according to the appropriateness, feasibility and the available resources
- seek and gain acceptance for the chosen strategy
- prepare long- and short-term plans to support and carry out the strategy
- implement the plan and conduct an ongoing evaluation of the situation as it evolves.

A similar process is graphically illustrated in Figure 7.1: the method of implementation required for the implementation of such a plan is answered in Rudyard Kiplings verse "The Elephant's Child":

> "I keep six honest serving men
> (They taught me all I know);
> Their names are WHAT and WHY and WHEN
> And HOW and WHERE and WHO."

In other words, the process is one determined by deciding: Who does what for whom? In what order and when? With what resources?

FIGURE 7.1: Strategic planning stage

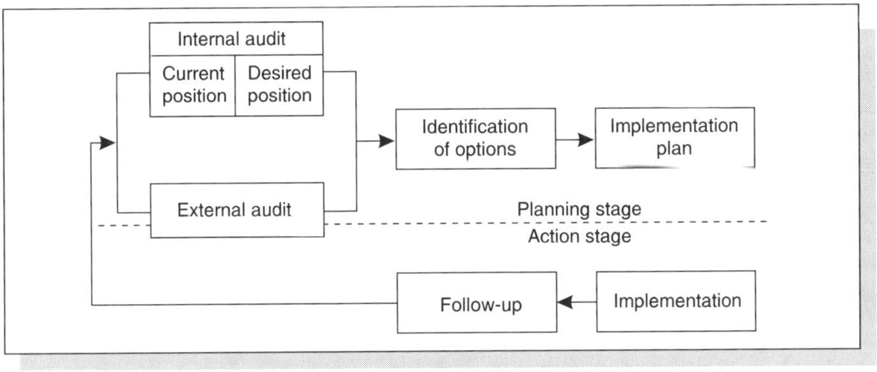

Source: Spiegal and Hyman (1991:6)

The Mosaic Strategic System Network developed by Scotti (1988) summarises the process of strategic planning (Figure 7.2).

FIGURE 7.2: Mosaic strategic system network

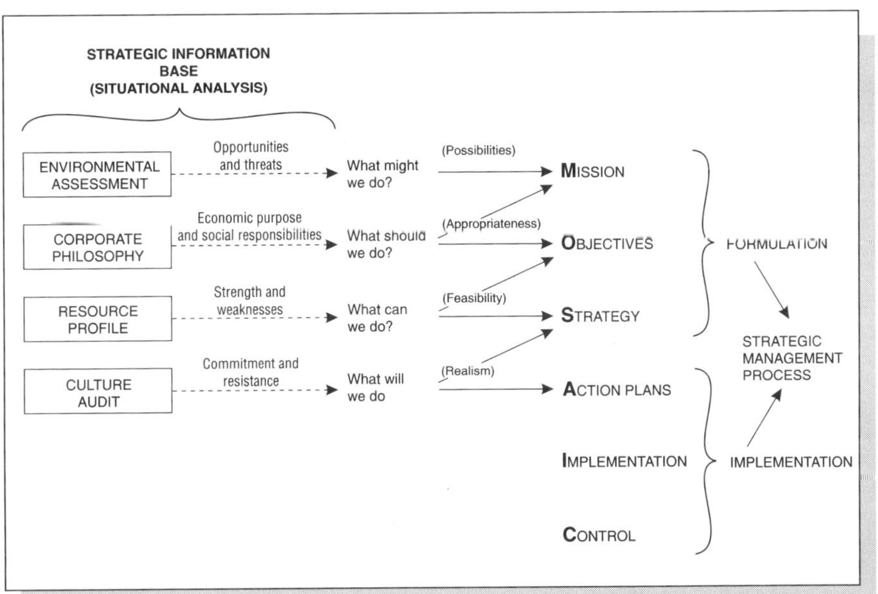

For a strategy or plan to be successful, the process must be placed within a time frame; that is, monitored and evaluated as part of the ongoing process. The success of any strategic plan is determined by measuring the impact of the implemented plans, outcomes of programmes, and the attainment of the identified goals and objectives.

The White Paper for the Transformation of the Health System of South Africa (Republic of South Africa 1997:1) "presents various implementation strategies designed to meet the basic needs of all our people, given the limited resources available." These strategies are found at the end of each chapter or health issue discussed in the document. Many of these strategies and others found in health policies and legislation, will be discussed further in this chapter.

7.4 POLICIES AND LEGISLATION

A policy is a course or principle of action, which provides guidelines for decision-making. Policies promote consistency in management decisions, while offering approaches which can be adapted to accommodate the different circumstances found in specific situations, regions, areas or communities. The health sector has undergone many changes since 1994 and many policies that directly affect or impact on health have been developed in collaboration with appropriate consultants, as well as the relevant role-players and stakeholders.

The policy of a country reflects the political will of the government in power. Health policy which influences the health and disease profile of the land, is therefore determined to a large extent by the level of importance that the government in power places on health, as well as the percentage of the national budget the government allocates to health. According to Draper (1991: 249), healthy political policy is dependent on "... political creativity and accountability which cannot be achieved without healthy democratic practices."

7.4.1 Legislation

Legislation is generated by stipulated competent authorities within a country. Legislation includes:

- *Statutes enacted by Parliament* - Statutory law (legislation) is the most important source of law in South Africa. The following statutes or Acts of Parliament are of special importance to health care:
  - *Constitution of the Republic of South Africa (Act 200 of 1993)*
  - *National Policy for Health Act, 116 of 1990*
  - *Health Act, 63 of 1977*
  - *International Health Regulation Act, 28 of 1974*
  - *Medicine and Related Substance Control Act, 101 of 1965*
  - *Hazardous Substance Act, 15 of 1973*
  - *Occupational Health and Safety Act, 85 of 1993*

  - *Mineral Act, 50 of 1991*
  - *Occupational Diseases in Mines and Works Act, 78 of 1973*
  - *Compensation for Occupational Injuries and Diseases Act, 130 of 1993*
  - *Unemployment Insurance Act, 30 of 1966*
  - *Labour Relations Act, 66 of 1995*
  - *Basic Conditions of Employment Act, 3 of 1983*
  - *Tobacco Produce Control Act, 83 of 1993*
  - *Atmospheric Pollution Prevention Act, 45 of 1965*
- *Subordinate legislation* - This term refers to:
  - Legislation established by the provinces in terms of the Constitution (previously referred to as ordinances).
  - Measures enacted by subsidiary legislative bodies such as Regional Service Councils and Local Authorities.
  - Regulations and proclamations that are enacted by the President or the relevant Minister in terms of an Act.
- *Impure law* - Statutory bodies such as the S A Nursing Council and the SA Medical and Dental Council are empowered to take decisions that have the same binding agreement as a law.

Both policies and legislation are implementation strategies. Policies are developed to guide the role-players in their endeavour to implement a strategy. Legislation, on the other hand, is more prescriptive as to the actual process of implementing a strategy - in other words, legislation is the legal basis whereby many policies are implemented. Statutes also have an enabling function, in that the legislation sets out the legal framework within which the relevant health team members may legally function.

The dilemma faced by the Ministry of Health in South Africa at the time of transformation, was how to take on the challenges of introducing new health policy, while continuing to work at, and contain, long-standing health-related problems. To determine this policy, a process of consultation was embarked upon with health committees and forums convened by the Ministry of Health, the provinces and various specialist groups. To obtain an even wider input, policies were also circulated to relevant stakeholders for comment, before they were finalised.

Many problems that have occurred in reorganising the health services for primary health care, have resulted from the absence of the comprehensive legislative framework that is required for the transformation. For example, the *Health Act* of 1977 is still legally enforceable and the implementation of a comprehensive primary health care service based on the district health system is not given the legal authority necessary to implement such a service.

Some of the new legislation that has impacted on health care includes the following:

(a) Constitution of the Republic of South Africa (Act 200 of 1993) as amended by Act 108 of 1996

The Constitution was prepared to provide South Africa with a legislative basis for the period of transition from apartheid to a democracy, and to entrench the democratic rights of all the people in South Africa. It was prepared from a political and juristic perspective. Certain aspects of the Constitution will have an impact on the health of all South Africans. Perhaps the most important contribution to the health of all South Africans, is that all people are now regarded as equal before the law, which is the basis of equity in health care.

The Bill of Rights is the cornerstone of democracy in South Africa. It enshrines the rights of all people in our country and affirms the democratic values of human dignity, equality and freedom. Specific individual rights are dealt with in Chapter 2 of the Act, Sections 7 to 33.

Section 27 deals specifically with health care, food, water and social security. It states that everyone has the right to have access to:

- health care services, including reproductive health care
- sufficient food and water
- social security, including appropriate social assistance, for people unable to support themselves and their dependants
- emergency medical treatment.

To achieve the progressive realisation of each of these rights, the State will need to introduce the necessary legislature and other appropriate measures, within its available resources. Other rights that can have a direct or indirect impact on health, are the right:

- to life
- to respect for and the protection of dignity
- to privacy
- to an environment that is not harmful to anyone's health and well-being
- to have access to adequate housing
- to fair labour practices including the right to join a trade union and to strike
- of children to basic nutrition, shelter, basic health services and social services.

These rights make it possible, in principle, for individuals and groups to demand certain basic health care services and a environment that is not harmful to their health and well-being, and to challenge the government when these are not provided.

The health worker may now join a trade union or other collective bargaining group, and strike if satisfaction is not obtained. However, the right of health workers can be challenged if the rights of individuals are threatened, e.g. the right of children to basic health services.

The section that pertains to the provision of health services states that the provision of health care is to be given by the three tiers of government. The Constitution contains information about these different levels of government - the national, provincial and local government - the latter are also referred to as municipalities. However, the Constitution does not clarify the role of the national level of government in health, and it refers to a local level of government; while government health policies mention the district level as the third tier of government. The role of the private sector in health care is also not clearly defined in the Constitution. All of these are aspects that can impact on the delivery of health care.

(b) The Choice on Termination of Pregnancy (TOP) Act (92 of 1996)

The path that this controversial Bill took from policy to legislation was a full two years, and a further three months before it could be implemented. The Act provides a legal framework through which women can exercise their constitutional right to reproductive choices. For the first time in South African history, women are able to request and give consent to an abortion, in the first twelve weeks of pregnancy.

Problems have occurred with the implementation of this Act at provincial level. The services do not have the facilities or the resources required to implement the legislation or to meet the demands of women who require this service.

Statistics indicate that in the first three months after the implementation of the Act, 7 300 abortions were performed, mostly in Gauteng province (Health Systems Trust 1997:147). Other problems encountered with the implementation of the Act, include those that relate to the moral dilemma that many service providers have in referring clients to such services and also in providing the termination of pregnancy service.

(c) The Medicine and Related Substance Control Amendment Act (90 of 1997)

This Amendment Bill was drafted and enacted to bring about the *Medicine and Related Substance Control Act* (101 of 1965) to enable the National Drug Policy to be implemented. The public generally accepted the National Drug Policy, but the reaction to the Bill was mixed, with wide criticism of the wording and the content. Concerns were raised by the pharmaceutical industry about the importation of parallel drugs which could have a negative economic effect on the industry.

The Act also deals with legalising and promoting the dispensing of generically equivalent medicines. Concern has been expressed on the proposed licensing of health professionals. Allowance is made for medical practitioners and nurses to dispense if licensed to do so by the Director-General, but the process and criteria for issuing the necessary licences are not stipulated in the Act. It is felt that aspects of the above legislation can impact negatively on the ability to use the skills and expertise that health professionals have available to implement the new health system, and therefore the legislation could limit the benefits of the new health dispensation and the positive effect it could bring to the people at ground level.

(d) The Nursing Amendment Act (19 of 1997)

This Bill was passed by the National Assembly in June 1997. The objective of this Nursing Amendment Bill was to enable the democratic election of a new Nursing Council. The proposed amendments to the Act were controversial and drew strong criticism from the nursing profession as well as from members of the public. The Portfolio Committee on Health amended the Act by increasing the number of nursing assistants, nursing auxiliary nurses, student nurses and community representatives on the Council. As a result of these amendments, professional nurses may not have the majority of seats in the Council. Since this body is responsible for the regulation and setting of standards for the nursing profession, the Bill met with antagonism. Further amendments were made to include a medical practitioner and a lawyer on the Council before the legislation was eventually passed. However, some antagonism still exists regarding the consultation process used concerning this legislation, and the position of nurses within the health system. Council elections have taken place, and the first meeting of the democratically elected SA Nursing Council was held in May 1998.

The implication of Section 38 of this Act is cause for concern to nurses. Conditions laid down in the Act, acknowledge the registered nurses' skills only under certain conditions, which are to the benefit of public services and other health professionals, rather than the registered nurses and the people whom they serve. The Act authorises registered nurses to:

- physically examine any person
- diagnose any physical defect, illness or deficiency in any person,
- keep prescribed medicine and supply, administer or prescribe
- promote family planning; but only under certain conditions.

The Act states that only those registered nurses who are in the employ of public health services and those designated by the Director-General are permitted to use the skills mentioned above. On a point of equity, this is of concern, since it can exclude all the nurses offering primary care services within the private sector. This will have an impact on the occupational health nurse, the private nurse practitioner, nurses working in multidisciplinary group practices which involve community health nurses, pharmacists and doctors, as well as those nurses in the employ of many non-governmental organisations, such as SANTA and the Hospice Association.

Further conditions of practice are applied to the nurse by the Act which states

> "... Provided that such (a) nurse may perform such act(s) only whenever the services of a medical practitioners or pharmacist , as the circumstances may require, are not available."

The motivation that was given, namely that these changes were effected to reflect the current health service system, does not hold true. Registered nurses offering these services are doing so in areas where doctors and pharmacists are available, but where the services required by the community exceed those that can be offered by the available doctor and/or pharmacist. Nurses functioning in this milieu will be able to increase the efficiency of such services by doing both the screening and treating of common conditions, enabling the doctor/pharmacist to fulfil the more complex medical role he or she is trained to do, in the interests of a more effective and efficient health service. The implications of this section of the Act are that it does not promote the optimal use of the available human resources in health service delivery.

(e) The Medical Dental and Supplementary Health Services Professions Amendment Act (1 of 1998)

The Act amends the Medical, Dental and Supplementary Health Professions Act of 1974, to make provision for the establishment of a Health Professions Council of South Africa, which will become the permanent statutory Health Professions Council to oversee the majority of the health professions. The structure of the new proposed Council is to be more representative of the member health professions than previously, when the Council focused mainly on the medical and dental professions. Provision is made within the Act for the establishment of professional boards for the various health professions, as well as for the representation of community nominees. Training regulation requirements and disciplinary powers would be devolved to the appropriate professional board.

Aspects of this legislation that were controversial and which were not adequately resolved, were related to the issuing of licenses to health professionals in order that they may dispense medicines, and the provision that made the Director-General responsible for this licensing.

Another issue which provoked a lot of debate at this time, and which was eventually excluded from this Act, was the two-year vocational training period proposed for doctors by the SAMDC. This period of compulsory training was to be implemented in January 1998, but has been put on hold and will probably be replaced by a one-year mandatory community service for doctors to be introduced sometime in the future. Concern has been expressed that the Department of National Health does not have the available resources or the necessary infrastructure to implement such a plan to the benefit of the community and the participating doctor.

(f) The Pharmacy Amendment Act (88 of 1997)

The Act proposed significant changes that would impact on pharmaceutical practice. Pharmacies may now be owned by people other than pharmacists as long as the pharmacy is under the constant supervision of a pharmacist. Pharmaceutical practice determined by the Act allows pharmacists more scope to function as members of the multidisciplinary health team at the community level, making them more valuable members of the team who implement primary health care. However, members of this discipline expressed their displeasure at the licensing procedure determined by the Act.

It was interesting to note that community representation is not required for this Council as is required by the legislation that governs the Health Professionals Council and the Nursing Council.

(g) The Draft Health Bill

The 9th draft of the National Health Bill was made available for comment in November 1996 and the promulgation of the new *National Health Act* was expected by the end of 1997. However this has not occurred, and in April 1997 the White Paper on the Transformation of the Health System in South Africa was published by the Ministry of Health. This document gives a comprehensive vision for the development of "... a unified health system capable of delivering quality health care to all our citizens efficiently and in a caring environment" (The Republic of South Africa 1997:5). No clarity has been forthcoming as to how this White Paper relates to the Draft Health Bill, however, and the strategies discussed in this document are dealt with very broadly and without time frames.

The continued absence of the new Health Act is of concern, since without the enabling legislative framework, it is not clear how the Department of Health will implement many of its new policies. This problem is further exacerbated by the conflicting legislation that is still in place from the previous government.

(h) Provincial Health Legislation

To date virtually no legislation has been passed by the nine provincial legislatures since they were established in 1994. The two provincial Acts that have been passed, are the *Hospital Act* of 1996 in the Free State, and the *Health, Developmental Social Welfare and Hospital Governance Act* of 1997 in the North West Province. Neither impact greatly on the implementation of primary health care (Health Systems Trust 1997:34) .

7.4.2 Health policies

Policy-making is a function of the Department of National Health and the implementation of policies is a function of the provinces. Policies are developed, based on information or research findings, and are implemented according to given guidelines. Most of the policies discussed below have been introduced since the 1994 elections.

Perhaps the most important guiding principles of the policies and strategies that have emanated from the Department of National Health during this period, have been about achieving greater equity in health care in South Africa and making services accessible to all. Some of the more important policies will be discussed in this section.

(a) Reconstruction and Development Programme (RDP)

In 1994 the Government of National Unity introduced a socio-economic development programme to ". . . mobilise all our people and our country's resources toward the final eradication of apartheid and the building of a democratic and non-sexist future" (ANC 1994(b):1). The Reconstruction and Development Programme aimed, through generating policies and implementing development programmes, to impact positively on the health status of the South African people. To initiate this process, a separate RDP Department was established in 1994 to identify areas where development programmes could be implemented to the benefit of communities. These programmes aimed at improving the total environment of a community, by introducing improvements to the infrastructure such as safe water projects, the building of clinics and schools, or by initiating projects that offered opportunities for employment, adult education and self-improvement. Another objective of such programmes was to empower people by involving them in their own development. There are six (6) basic principles that make up the political and economic philosophy that underlie the RDP, namely that the programme must:

- be an integrated and sustainable programme

- be a people-driven process
- promote peace and security
- form the basis of nation-building
- link reconstruction and development
- form part of the democratisation of South Africa.

The closure of the RDP offices in March 1996 was seen by many as the abandonment of the socio-economic or integrated approach to development, which is an important part of comprehensive primary health care. However, this was not necessarily the case and the functions of the RDP office were devolved to each of the appropriate departments, who then took the responsibility for the promotion, funding and implementation of development programmes that impacted on that particular department. It is, however, difficult to implement such programmes without intersectoral collaboration, as is illustrated in the path model illustrated in Figure 7.3.

FIGURE 7.3: A path model of the effects of investment in water and sanitation

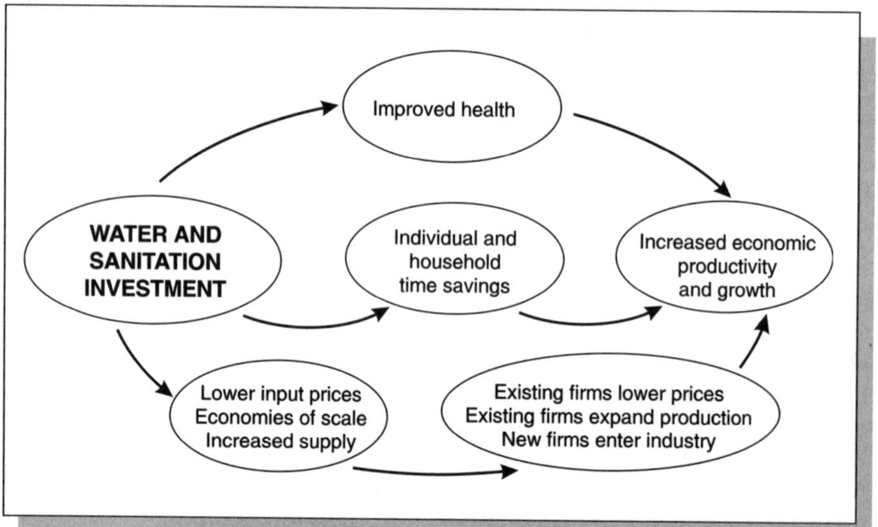

Source: Health Systems Trust (1996:16)

Adequate housing is essential for attaining optimal health. The development of a National Housing Strategy, which was formulated and negotiated with all the relevant stakeholders and which was accepted at the Botshabelo Housing Summit, formed the basis of the programme. Provincial Housing Boards have been established and funding has been made available. However, despite all the necessary components for the programme being in place, the number of houses actually built has fallen far short of the number required, and this has resulted in people becoming frustrated and angry because their expectations have not been met. Informal housing settlements have developed rapidly in most urban areas and this has impacted negatively on health.

By contrast, the provision of clean water to communities has been one of the most visible and successful initiatives of the government development programme. Eskom's electrification programme has also been successful and the number of new connections has increased four times in the last four years. These initiatives have been associated with the decline in morbidity rates in certain areas.

The Mashakane campaign was introduced to improve service delivery and to increase the payment for services rendered by the user. The campaign was patronised by President Nelson Mandela, and has had good effect in some areas, and virtually no effect in others.

Several other initiatives have been introduced since then, the most significant being the macro-economic strategy of Growth, Employment and Redistribution (GEAR), which is intended to provide opportunities for employment and to reduce the problem of poverty in this country.

(b) Traditional healers

Traditional medicine is defined by the World Health Organisation (WHO) as:

> "Comprising therapeutic practices that have been in existence, often for hundreds of years, before the development and spread of modern scientific medicine and are still in use today. These practices vary widely, in keeping with the social and cultural heritage of different countries."

The WHO supports a realistic, pragmatic approach to the traditional healer for the following reasons:

- The greatest part of the world's population relies on traditional medicine which has the potential for playing an important role in primary health care.
- Medicinal plants are important in the lives of individuals and communities. Research and exchange of information from a conservation perspective, as well as the utilisation of these medicinal plants in health care, is essential.

The WHO therefore supports the formulation of national policy and the evaluation of traditional practices, including the safety and efficiency of traditional medicines. It is also important to upgrade the knowledge and skills of traditional healers and to inform and educate the community regarding their role.

As far as current policy that is being developed in South Africa with regard to traditional medicine is concerned, discussions over a period of time between the Department of Health and various traditional healer organisations, culminated in the establishment of an Interim Committee for Traditional Healers during 1992. In 1993, a National Steering Committee for Traditional Healers (NASCOTH), consisting of 10 members, was elected.

The Department of Health recognises that traditional healers have a role to play in health care and has initiated the following investigations and programmes to accomplish this.

- The Executive Council of Health has been requested by the Minister of Health to investigate possible ways to register traditional healers. At present (1998) KwaZulu-Natal is licensing traditional healers.
- A Human Resources Development Committee was appointed by the Minister of Health to develop a draft policy regarding the whole spectrum of human resources in health care, as well as to examine the role of traditional healers in a new health service dispensation.
- Training programmes for traditional healers have been developed by the Department of National Health. These cover topics such as HIV-AIDS, mental health, rehydration programmes, cancer treatment, tuberculosis and aspects of maternal and child health care.

Traditional birth attendants (TBAs) are also seen as part of the traditional healer cadre and they are working closely with registered midwives in some rural areas. To date a policy document has not been made available.

(c) Maternal, Child and Women's Health Policy

Maternal and child health care is one of the essential components of comprehensive primary health care. In 1995 the Maternal, Child and Women's Health Plan (MCWH) was developed and the South African government became a signatory to the Convention of the Rights of the Child. Soon after this the Government of National Unity announced free health care for mothers and children under the age of six (6) years and the introduction of a primary school nutrition programme.

The Beijing Women's Conference was held by the United Nations in September 1995. The focus of the conference was on practical ways to implement women's full and equal partnerships in development, politics, decision-making, and in international co-operation to achieve world peace. The South African government committed itself to adoption of all parts of the platform of action. The Conference gave greater clarity to the policy issues in relation to women's health.

Priority health problems for women that need to be urgently addressed in

South Africa, include HIV/AIDS, sexually-transmitted diseases and carcinoma of the cervix. Violence against women is also an escalating problem which is of concern.

In 1995 the infant mortality rate (IMR) for black children in South Africa was between 30 and 73 per 1 000 live births, which was as much as seven times higher than children from other population groups in this country (Health Systems Trust 1996:173). Good antenatal, delivery and postnatal care is needed to reduce this very high mortality rate.

The most important causes of mortality and morbidity in infants and young children were conditions such as malnutrition and infections such as diarrhoeal diseases and acute respiratory conditions. The HIV/AIDS problem is a rapidly increasing threat to children's health. The number of AIDS orphans is increasing and these will require more and more support from the State, but care will have to be community-based. The term "child" refers to anybody under the age of 18, in accordance with the Convention on the Rights of the Child.

Through implementing the WHO Expanded Programme of Immunisation (EPI) in April 1995, it is hoped to achieve a 95% immunisation coverage by the year 2000. In 1995 the polio vaccination campaign reached almost 90% of the targeted children and in 1996 the polio vaccination campaign was repeated, together with a measles vaccination campaign. Problems in maintaining the cold chain, especially in rural areas, will have to be addressed if these objectives are to be met. It is the aim of the Health Ministry to declare South Africa to be polio-free early in the next century.

The implementation of the MCWH policy has generally been slower than anticipated, mainly due to the lack of the necessary resources. The introduction of free services resulted in increased attendance at public health facilities by both pregnant women and children under six. Where facilities lacked the resources or these were inadequate and they were unable to cope with the demands made, the second and third levels of facilities were swamped and overextended to meet the needs of the people. This has resulted in an often frustrated and demotivated workforce.

(d) The National Drug Policy

The National Drug Policy (NDP) was launched in February 1996. The drug policy is an integral part of the National Health Policy which aims at equity in the provision of health care for all.

The goal of the NDP is to ensure an adequate and reliable supply of safe, cost-effective drugs of acceptable quality to all citizens of South Africa and the rational use of drugs by prescribers, dispensers and consumers (DOH 1996:3).

Essential drugs are mentioned in the document, and these refer to drugs that are required to treat the majority of conditions that are prevalent in a country in a cost-effective and efficient manner. They comprise the drugs most needed for the health care of the majority of the population which must be available and accessible to all citizens at all times (DOH 1996:4) .

A South African Essential Drug List which will contain approximately 200 generic drugs, was drawn up in consultation with role-players from all the different disciplines and was published in April 1996. The generic name of the drug is also referred to as the non-proprietary name or a name that pertains to what the drug contains rather than the name given by a specific company and under which the drug is marketed.

This document offers guidelines to health care providers about how the policy can be implemented. Key issues in the policy are:

- *Medicine Control Council (MCC)*: The Council will be strengthened to enable it to review the appropriate legislation and regulations to support the objectives of the NDP. Another function of this council will be to fund drug evaluation and testing to ensure safe drugs, as well as to liaise with the relevant departments and organisations to ensure the implementation of the policy. Recently the Minister of Health has disbanded this statutory body and is in the process of developing another alternative body to take on these duties.
- *Registration or licensing of practitioners and premises*: The policy states that medical practitioners and nurses will not be permitted to dispense drugs, except where separate pharmaceutical services are not available. Where doctors and nurses do dispense, these persons must be in possession of a dispensing license which will be issued by the MCC. Special concessions will be granted to occupational health services, but the policy does not elaborate on what these concessions are. It also refers to proven competency of these practitioners to dispense drugs by virtue of the successful completion of a suitable training programme(DOH 1996:6).

Premises where dispensing occurs must be registered and/or licensed in terms of the *Medicine and Related Substance Control Act* (101 of 1965). These premises will be subject to inspection by the provincial authorities on guidelines drawn up by the MCC (DOH 1996:6).

The Department of Health issued permits to registered nurses and pharmacists in terms of the *Medicine and Related Substance Control Amendment Act* 101 of 1965, which read as follows:

> "Notwithstanding the other provisions of this section, the Director-General may, after consultation with the Pharmacy Board, issue a permit to any person or organisation performing a health service, authorising such a person or organisation to acquire, possess, use or supply any specific Schedule 1, Schedule 2,

Schedule 3 or Schedule 4 substance, and such a permit will be subject to such conditions as Director-General may determine."

However, the regulations which should specify the circumstances under which such permits are issued have not been formulated. Until this policy is implemented no permits are being issued by the Department of Health.

- *Rationalisation of the drug pricing and selection*: The policy advocates that all drugs at the primary care level will be free of charge. At secondary and tertiary level an affordable fee will be levied. The use of generic drugs is recommended to reduce drug costs. Incentives will be introduced that should favour generic drugs and their production in South Africa. Prescriptions must be written using these approved generic names and until this is achieved, generic substitution will be allowed through legislation. A list of products that cannot be substituted will be prepared and disseminated by the MCC (DOH 1996:9).
- *A national essential drug list*: An essential drug list using generic names will be drawn up and reviewed every two years. The National Essential Drug List Committee is a multidisciplinary group appointed by the Minister of Health to draw up this list and to develop standard treatment guidelines (DOH 1996). It is presently being revised and should be available by the end of 1998.
- *Storage and safeguarding of drugs*: Standard Operating Procedures (SOPs) have been developed and will be updated regularly. They will include practical guidelines to cover all administrative procedures to manage and control the storage and distribution of drugs and medical supplies. Methods of defining maximum and minimum stock levels will also be suggested, as well as guidelines on systematic stock rotation and the handling of obsolete and expired stock. (DOH 1996:12–13)
- *Rational drug use*: Through the adequate training of health personnel involved in diagnosis, and prescribing and dispensing drugs, it is hoped to achieve the informed and appropriate use of drugs in the community.

The DOH will be responsible for the dissemination of information to prescribers and dispensers. Drug Information Centres will be established, and regularly updated protocols for the treatment of common conditions with essential drugs and an annual national formulary of essential drugs will be distributed (DOH 1996:16–17).

(e) The Population Policy

A draft White Paper for a Population Policy appeared in the *Government Gazette* on 31 October 1996. The vision of the policy emphasises the attainment of a high and equitable quality of life for South Africans, and forms part of the national development strategy. It acknowledges that population, development and the environment are intricately interrelated.

(f) The National Health Information System (NHISSA)

The lack of reliable health information is a major obstacle to effective planning in health care. It also inhibits the ability to assess the effectiveness of implemented health programmes. In 1994 the Minister of Health established a committee of stakeholders to determine this policy.

The existing information systems were fragmented and often incompatible. In 1995 Dr SH Mandil, a WHO Advisor on Informatics, acted as Principal Consultant for the development of NHISSA at the request of the Health Minister. He headed a committee that consisted of representatives from all the provinces, the Department of Health, the Medical Research Council, universities and members from the private sector (WHO 1995:6). The determined objectives of the NHISSA are to:

- ensure the availability of information for the effective planning and management of health services at all levels
- measure the health status of the South African population
- monitor and measure the progress of developmental priorities.

To capture data from health facilities at community level, the Regional Health Management Information Service (RHMIS) is being used. It is a health management system that captures data from all health facilities, both private and public, and uses standard national definitions so that information is comparable across regions and provinces.

7.5 MANAGEMENT DEVELOPMENT FOR PRIMARY HEALTH CARE

In many countries worldwide, weak management is often cited as the reason for the failure to implement primary health care. Other aspects that impact on implementation that are often raised, are the need to effectively decentralise health care and to strengthen district or local health systems.

To bridge the gap between policy and the implementation of primary health care requires good management skills. Concern has been expressed by the WHO, that although many countries have directed a considerable amount of their limited resources to management training, the results have been disappointing. In May 1990 the WHO (WHO 1990(b):1) organised a meeting of consultants to discuss this problem and to identify ways in which health management development could improve the implementation of primary health care programmes.

They found that many of the problems found in implementing primary health care are due to a lack of skills, resources, information, unclear procedures of operation and poorly motivated staff.

Other problems found in implementing primary health strategies include the existing organisational structures and the systems through which strategies are to be implemented. There is often a mismatch between strategy and structure. If there is a mismatch, the structure with the management system will need to be changed, or the strategy will need to be questioned and reassessed. Therefore to implement primary health care as a strategy, there is often a need to make the structural changes that are necessary to facilitate the process.

There is a need for the management development for primary health care to be concerned with improving

> "... implementation within the constraints of existing structures and systems and also with changing structures and systems in relation to primary health care policies" (WHO 1990(b):7).

Nurses in South Africa constitute 67,8% of all health workers. There are more than 160 000 nurses of all categories, which gives an acceptable ratio of nurses to population. However, the maldistribution of nursing staff between urban and rural areas is evident (Bierman 1994:141), with some rural areas having virtually no health workers at all.

The nurse is the member of the health team who is the most universally involved in primary health care and, because of the dynamic nature of nursing, has often filled in for other health professionals when these are not available. She plays a key role as a co-ordinator or facilitator of the health care team and as an independent accountable practitioner. However, legal limitations are encountered in practice, in that the nurse who must often practise in relative isolation, may not prescribe medicines unless authorised to do so in terms of section 38a of the *Nursing Act* of 1978 (as amended).

Nursing education has traditionally centred on curative, hospital-based care and is dominated by the medical model. A shift has occurred in basic professional education to a more community-orientated approach but it has not been sufficient to prepare nurses adequately for primary health care.

To meet the primary health care needs of the community, education needs to be based on the health model, with community-based learning and the community as client. The skills required will go beyond the traditional scope of nursing and require more interdisciplinary training and interaction. Registered nurses should have these skills and the qualification of community nurse should be developed to meet the more specialised needs of community practice.

However, post-basic courses and in-service training being offered are emphasising the curative aspect of primary health care: the diagnosis and treatment of individuals with minor ailments rather than the preventive and promotive community-based care, in other words, comprehensive primary health care. The nurses who have attended these courses are often referred to as primary health care nurses. This approach is limiting the vital role which nurses should and could be playing in the South African health system.

7.6 DISTRICT HEALTH SERVICES

In 1986 the WHO Global Programme Committee defined the District Health System as follows:

> "A district health system based on primary health care, is a more or less self-contained segment of the national health system. It comprises first and foremost a well defined population, living within a clearly delineated administrative and geographical area, whether urban or rural. It includes all institutions and individuals providing health care in the district, whether governmental, social security, non-governmental, private or traditional. A district health system, therefore, consists of a large variety of interrelated elements that contribute to health in homes, schools, work places, and communities, through the health and other related sectors. It includes self care and all health care workers and facilities, up to and including the hospital at the first referral level and the appropriate laboratory, other diagnostic and logistic support services. Its component elements need to be well co-ordinated by an officer assigned to this function in order to draw together all these elements and institutions into a fully comprehensive range of promotive, preventive, curative and rehabilitative health activities" (WHO 1988:9).

7.6.1 An overview of the district health system

According to the WHO (1988:9), a district health system is based on the Declaration of Alma-Ata and on the global strategy of health for all, and should incorporate the following general principles:

- equity
- accessibility
- emphasis on health promotion and prevention
- intersectoral action
- community involvement
- decentralisation
- the integration of health programmes
- co-ordination of separate health activities.

The term "district" is used in a generic sense and denotes an area that is clearly defined both geographically and administratively. The population is usually between 50 000 and 500 000, has some form of local government and it should have a hospital for referral support. The organisation and structure of the district will be developed according to each specific country's needs and situation.

The district is the most appropriate level to co-ordinate top-down and bottom-up planning for primary health care. It is also the level where the community can be involved in the planning and implementation of primary health care programmes. Since most community development occurs at this level, intersectoral co-operation must also be facilitated here.

The responsibility for promoting, implementing and supporting primary health care falls to district management. For the process to be successful, the management skills of these health workers will need to be developed. The aspects that will require urgent attention if district health systems are to function, are referred to as the main pillars of the district health system. They include:

- organisation, planning and management
- financing and resource allocation
- intersectoral action
- community involvement
- development of human resources.

For districts to function effectively, there must be a national policy, and the system must have both the commitment and the support of the national level of government. Through the process of decentralisation, sufficient authority in decision-making, as well as resource allocation, must be delegated to the district manager for effective planning and management to occur at this level.

7.6.2 Health care in South Africa

The government's core functions in health, and at all levels of government, are assessment, policy development and assurance. In addition to these functions, which are the responsibility of the national, provincial and district levels of government, each level has unique responsibilities.

The three levels of responsibility in South African government will be discussed below as their functions are interrelated. The levels are:

- *The national level* – The Department of Health is the central force in public health and must bear ultimate responsibility for the health of the nation. Since taking office it has fulfilled its task to ". . . develop guidelines, norms and standards to apply throughout the health system, as was stated in the ANC National Health Plan" (ANC 1994(a):68).

  A committee of inquiry into a national health insurance system was set up and produced a report – *Restructuring the National Health System for universal primary health care*. The report recommended, among other things, that a target be set for five years to attain universal access to primary health care for all South Africans, that free health care be made available for all, but that the choice remains for individuals to belong to private medical schemes and medical insurance (Broomberg and Shisana 1995:1–11). This has impacted on the other levels of delivery, especially the local or district level, since demands on services have increased and the infrastructure and resources have not been available to meet these demands.

- *The provincial level* – The rationale was that provincial health departments would take control of all health services in the province, and that once district boundaries were in place, and managers suitably trained, power would be devolved to the districts.

  All provinces have been divided into regions to assist with administration. In some provinces the departments administer health and welfare, and in others just health. This does lead to some confusion and difficulty since directives from the Department of Health come from two different departments. Sufficient authority in decision-making and resource allocation needs to be delegated to the district manager for effective planning and management to occur at district level. The mechanism by which this is to be achieved must still be determined.
- *District level* – The policy for the development of a District Health System for South Africa was published and circulated for public comment in December 1995. The policy developed is based on the premise that the district must be large enough to be economically efficient and small enough to ensure effective management which is accountable to the local community (DOH 1995:3–5).

According to general guidelines issued by the Department of Health, a district health system is defined as comprising:

- a well-defined population living within a clearly delineated administrative and geographical area;
- all institutions and individuals providing health care within this district, including all health workers and facilities, up to and including hospitals at the first referral level, and the appropriate laboratory and other diagnostic and logistical support services.

Setting up boundaries for districts is in progress. In some provinces the districts have corresponded to one or more local authority boundaries and in others there is no correspondence at this stage (Health Systems Trust 1996:36).

The district is the foundation of the South African health system because it

FIGURE 7.4: Proposed organogram of the national health system at the district level

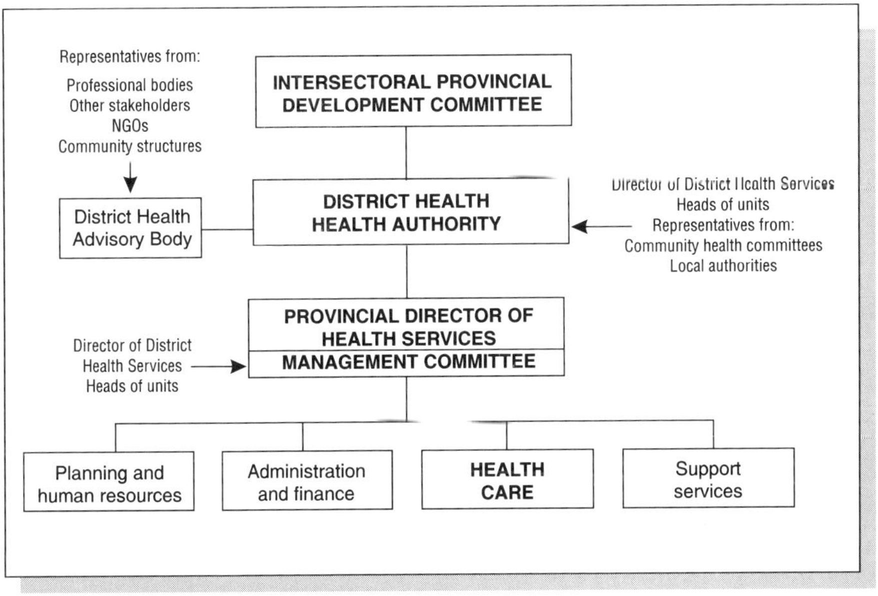

Source: ANC (1994:63)

is at this level that primary health care is implemented. However, this is the level where the least progress has been noted. The functioning of these services is being hampered by the following issues:

- the governance and management of the district system
- the relationship between state and local authorities
- the form of representation of local communities
- the disparity of salaries and conditions of service between these and "old" services in local authorities and provinces
- the relationship between districts and community hospitals, especially in urban areas (Health Systems Trust 1996:xiv).

The support system needed between the three levels of government to enable the health system to be functional, is represented in a simplified form in Figure 7.5 (DOH 1995:10).

7.7 SUMMARY

Twenty years after the introduction of the primary health care approach at Alma-Ata, many countries around the world are politically committed to implementing appropriate health systems to implement primary health care.

FIGURE 7.5: The support system between three levels of government

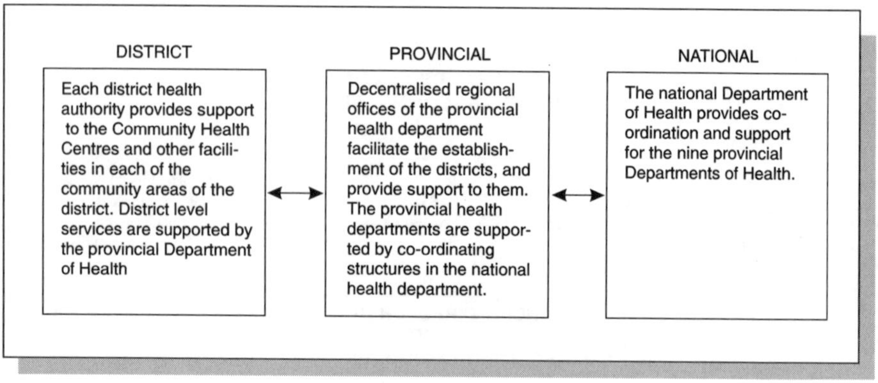

However, the promotion of healthy practices and the prevention of disease in communities continue to receive considerably less emphasis than the care of sick individuals who attend clinics or other health institutions seeking help. Considerable progress has been made in South Africa in improving and extending the coverage of health services, making them more accessible to people in the communities, although there is still a strong emphasis on medical or curative services. At community or district level, epidemiological methods are rarely used to assess the health status in the population or to identify problems that may need to take priority, and intersectoral approaches to health are not well co-ordinated to use the available resources more rationally. These issues will have to be dealt with if comprehensive primary health care is to really be successfully implemented and optimal health attained for all.

Bibliography

African National Congress. 1994(a). *A national health plan for South-Africa.* Johannesburg: ANC.

African National Congress. 1994(b). *The reconstruction and development programme.* Johannesburg : Unanyano.

Bierman, J. 1994. Legal limitations to primary health care practice in South Africa. *International journal of medicine and law.* Vol. 13, No. 1:141–153.

Broomberg, J. and Shisana, O. 1995. *Restructuring the national health system for universal primary health care.* Pretoria: Department of Health.

Clark, M.J. 1996. *Nursing in the community.* 2nd edition. Norwalk: Apple & Lange.

Department of Health. 1995. *A policy for the development of the district health system for South Africa.* Department of Health: Pretoria.

Department of Health. 1996. *National drug policy for South Africa.* CTP Book Printers: Cape Town.

Department of Welfare. 1996. *Draft white paper for a population policy.* Pretoria: Government Printer.

Draper, P. (Ed.) 1991. *Health through public policy. The greening of public health.* London: Green print.

Folscher, C.W. 1994. Nurses and Traditional Healers. Department of Health: Unpublished paper.

Gilbert, L., Selikow, T.A. and Walker, L. 1996. *Society, Health and Disease: An introductory reader for health professionals.* Randburg: Ravan.

Greef, M. 1990. Building blocks. *Nursing RSA Verpleging.* Vol. 5, No. 7:10–11.

Health Systems Trust and Henry J. Kaiser Family Foundation. 1996. *South African Health Review.* Durban: Fishwick Printers.

Health Systems Trust. 1997. *South African Health Review.* Durban: Kwik Kopy Printing.

Institute of Medicine. 1993. *The future of public health.* Washington: National Academy Press.

King, L.J. 1996. Community participation in health care delivery. Unpublished thesis. Pretoria: Unisa.

Moller, H. and Donohue, S. 1995. *Primary health care formulary.* Cape Town: CTP Printers.

Morley, D., Rhode, J. and Williams, G. 1989. *Practising health for all.* Oxford: Oxford University Press.

Nyasulu, N.D. and Mzolo, N.C. 1990. Traditional birth attendants in Brazil. *Nursing RSA Verpleging.* Vol. 8, No. 4:13–16.

Oskowitz, B. 1991. Bridging the communication gap between traditional healers and nurses. *Nursing RSA Verpleging.* Vol. 6, No. 7:20–21.

Report. 1996. *Beijing Conference: plan of action.* Johannesburg: Umanyano.

Republic of South Africa. 1990. *The Constitution of the Republic of South Africa.* Act 108 of 1996. Pretoria: Government Printer.

Republic of South Africa. 1997. White paper for the transformation of the health system in South Africa. Pretoria: Government Printer.

Spiegal, A.D. and Hyman, H.H. 1991. *Strategic health planning: methods and techniques applied to marketing and management.* Norwood: Ablex Publishing Corporation.

Spradley, B.W. and Allender, J.A. 1996. *Community health nursing. Concepts and practice.* 4th edition. Philadelphia: Lippencott.

Stanhope, M. and Lancaster, J. 1996. *Community health nursing. Promoting health of aggregates, families, and individuals.* 4th edition. St Louis: Mosby.

Swanson, J. M. and Albrecht, M. 1993. *Community health nursing. Promoting the health of aggregates.* Philadelphia: W.B. Saunders.

Troskie, R. 1995. *The role of the nurse in collaborating with traditional healers in primary health clinics*. UNISA: Unpublished research report.

World Health Organisation. 1978. *The promotion and development of traditional medicine*. (Technical report 622). Geneva: WHO.

World Health Organisation. 1988. *The challenge of implementation: District health services for primary health care*. Geneva: WHO.

World Health Organisation. 1990(a). *Improving urban health: Guidelines for rapid appraisal to assess community health needs*. Geneva: WHO.

World Health Organisation. 1990(b). *Management development for primary health care*. Geneva: WHO.

World Health Organisation. 1992. *A call for the new public health action*. Geneva: WHO.

World Health Organisation/EURO. 1994. *Training and research in public health: Policy perspectives for a "New public health"*. Karlstad: WHO Collaborating Centre.

World Health Organisation. 1995. *The national health information system of South Africa (NHISSA): from start to implementation*. Geneva: WHO.

Index